Medical Ethics
and Meaning at
End of Life

Richard George Boudreau

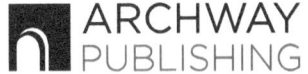
ARCHWAY
PUBLISHING

Archway Publishing books may be ordered through booksellers or by contacting:

Archway Publishing
1663 Liberty Drive
Bloomington, IN 47403
www.archwaypublishing.com
844-669-3957

ISBN: 978-1-6657-1371-9 (sc)
ISBN: 978-1-6657-1370-2 (hc)
ISBN: 978-1-6657-0743-5 (e)

Library of Congress Control Number: 2021920700

Print information available on the last page.

Archway Publishing rev. date: 11/23/2021

CONTENTS

CHAPTER 3
RESEARCH METHODS

ABSTRACT

As people age through the life span, many focus with increasing intensity on the issues they face as elderly members of society and as people facing end-of-life decision-making. The inevitability of death does not detract from the onset of death anxiety and conflicted views that emerge because of the range of impacts of aging. End-of-life issues, including fear of dying, have been recognized as a factor hindering psychosocial functioning in elderly populations. Subsequently, defining therapeutic methods through which individuals can address their fears and alleviate anxiety have become goals in creating dynamic psychotherapeutic approaches.

One of the emerging strategies outlined in the current literature is the use of existential philosophical principles in the creation of an operational psychoanalytic praxis. Because end-of-life issues often result in the desire by individuals to confront their existence (existential philosophy), the application of an existential psychotherapeutic approach has been introduced as a part of existing research. This has led to the identification of "death fear" as a major development in the presence of end-of-life assessments. An operational psychoanalytic model that addresses the issue of the fear of death has been identified as a major development in creating a workable psychoanalytic praxis.

The underlying belief shared by researchers is that fear is inherent for both doctors and patients and requires understanding and compassion on both sides of the equation. The implementation of a feasible psychoanalytical praxis that takes into consideration the benefits of an existential and "pathosophical" (empathy-based) approach to treatment is a necessary improvement to existing structures. This research study is designed to assess the models or psychoanalytical praxes introduced when addressing the needs of elderly individuals and to evaluate both the historical context in which they were formed and the support mechanisms for their continuation. Through a close scrutiny of existing approaches, the evidence presented supports the benefits of existential and pathosophical praxis to create responsive options for elderly patients seeking support at the end of life. The implementation and feasibility of suitable approaches must be guided by bedrock medical ethical principles, including beneficence, nonmaleficence, autonomy, veracity, dignity, and justice.

HISTORICAL EXISTENTIAL PERSPECTIVE

Galen (AD 129–200) was one of the most prominent ancient physicians as well as a philosopher. He was also a well-read scholar who combined extensive erudition with cutting-edge observational practice to completely change the understanding and teaching of medicine. He frequently integrated his observational practice with the natural philosophy of Plato and Aristotle. His position as the leading authority in medical theory extended for at least fourteen hundred years.

Galen correctly saw that there is a methodological difference between taking account of the patient in front of you in all of the patient's particularity and, instead, understanding the patient in front of you as representing an instance of a general rule of biomedical science. The way that Galen sought to insert himself into this debate makes his conclusions relevant to medicine today.

Before sickness came to be perceived primarily as an

organic or behavioral abnormality, he who got sick could still find in the eyes of the doctor a reflection of his own anguish and some recognition of the uniqueness of his suffering. Now what he meets is the gaze of a biological accountant engaged in input/output calculations. His sickness is taken from him and turned into the raw material for an institutional enterprise. His condition is interpreted according to a set of abstract rules in a language he cannot understand. He is taught only about alien entities that the doctor combats, but only just as much as the doctor considers necessary to gain the patient's cooperation. Language is taken over by the doctors; the sick person is deprived of meaningful words for his anguish, which is thus further increased by linguistic mystification.

Come forward to Ivan Illich (1926–2002), an Australian philosopher, Roman Catholic priest, and a "maverick social critic" of contemporary Western culture. He stated, "It is of the highest importance that there be thinking physicians, who are not of a mind to leave the field for the scientific technologists." What biological medicine or "biomedicine" can offer the patient is short- or long-term relief from pain and suffering, its long-term "management" or its substitution by other forms of pain and suffering (side effects, reduced quality of life, etc.). What it cannot and does not even seek to offer the patient is a way of managing to understand the meaning of that pain and suffering, not just as an expression of the life of their bodies or brains but as an embodiment of their life world as whole—with all its life dilemmas and distress, life pain, and life suffering.

Physical or mental pain and suffering are not just a natural part of life—rather than something that merely interferes with or obstructs our lives. In their very essence and origin, pain and suffering are an expression of our life and our existence or life world as a whole. Understood in this way, biological medicine has not begun to understand the true origin or "etiology" of illness, obsessed as it is with finding and treating its biological "causes" and failing completely to explore its life meaning, life purpose, and life origin. Nor has biomedicine begun to understand the very meaning of the term *biology* itself, which refers, in its Greek origins, to the "speech" *(logos)* of "life" *(bios)*. Only when the human body is understood as a living language of the human being, and illness as a form of bodily speech giving expression to the life of the human being, can "the essential realm in which biology moves"— our lives—come to life in "biology as a science." Only in this way too can we also learn to understand illness pathosophically, as suffering or pathos that is a pregnant source of life wisdom.

At the heart of this project for a new existential and "pathosophical" approach to medicine is a fundamental distinction between the body as perceived "externally" or "exteroceptively" (the so-called "physical" body) and the body as subjectively or "enterceptively" felt and experienced from within—the "felt body" or "lived body" (German Leib). Along with this distinction goes the recognition that all "psychic" phenomena, far from being reducible to products of the physical body and brain, are essentially experienced dimensions of the individual's lived body—itself an embodiment or "bodying forth" of the individual's entire existential life world and life history as a whole.

Heidegger stated, "Every feeling is an embodiment attuned in this or that way, a mood that embodies in this or that way." Put in other terms, every state of consciousness or "psychical" state is always and at the same time a felt bodily or "somatic" state—and vice versa. Or as Weizsäcker put it, "Nothing organic has no meaning; nothing psychical has no body."

It follows that a truly "phenomenological" and "existential" approach to health and illness must—in principle—challenge the entire social, cultural, economic, institutional, professional, and personal separation between "psychotherapy" in all its forms (including "existential psychotherapy") and "somatic" medicine. Indeed, "existential medicine" is, in its very essence, the abolition of this separation and in this sense may be described as marking "the end of psychotherapy and the rethinking of medicine." For to separate "psychological" *dis-ease* and therapies from bodily *dis-ease* and therapies is to deny the essence of medicine—of therapy as such.

An existential "rethinking of medicine" requires first of all a revelation of the root metaphysical assumptions and metaphors that shape the dominant biomedical model of health and illness—first and foremost the mechanistic assumption that illnesses have biological "causes" rather than existential meanings. Second is the basic military metaphor of "war" against diseases and death—whether fought through the medium of biomedical research or the body's own so-called immune "defenses." Here it is not enough to question such metaphysical assumptions and metaphors merely within the framework of a general "philosophy of medicine." Instead, what is needed is a critical examination and rethinking of specific biological sciences and their languages (e.g., the languages of genetics and molecular biology, immunology, virology, and oncology). This in turn is impossible without knowledge of both the philosophical roots and historical evolution of the biological sciences and their languages.

A thorough phenomenological rethinking of medicine must also address in a new way the nature and essence, not just of body hood as such but also the nature of specific organs, bodily functions, and their associated organic "disorders" or "diseases," thus enabling us to understand their complex and intricate "biology" in the root sense of this term—as an expression of the logos or "speech" of life (bios), something in no way reducible molecular-genetic alphabet and vocabulary.

Taking a cursory "medical history" of a patient without any interest in and attention to their life history cannot lead to genuine insight into the life of the patient's body, let alone awaken sensitivity to their lived body, something inseparable from their life and lived world. The cultivation of existential medicine as a practice must therefore above all address the question of what would constitute an existential-phenomenological analysis of specific medical conditions in the larger context of an individual patient's entire life world and life history—thus coming to more deeply know the patient as a human being through this knowing *(dia-gnosis)*. Here, careful and thoughtful existential analyses and case studies of individuals suffering—perhaps for quite different reasons—from specific biomedically defined and diagnosed diseases, such as diabetes or the varieties of cancer, are called for.

For the task of the purely biomedical physician is precisely not to think but rather to simply act—in accordance with their training and in strict conformity to a regulatory professional or institutional bureaucracy.

"Ours is not to reason why …" is the motto of biomedical practice, particularly if this includes the central question of illness per se: why this particular illness, and why now? No less important for the existential therapist—understood as an "existential physician" or "life doctor"—is the question of what would constitute an innately therapeutic relationship with the individual patient and how such a relational comportment can be cultivated. For this comportment must be one in which a phenomenological stance is not merely adopted as a theoretical position but can itself be actively embodied in ways that are in themselves therapeutic.

As regards the role of this particular site in addressing in pursuing and stimulating the overall project of recalling and rethinking the existential foundations of medicine, its aim is also to ensure a reasonable balance between content that is (a) accessible and of personal value to the "lay" reader and (b) of specific interest to readers familiar with fields, such as phenomenology and hermeneutics, psychoanalysis and Daseinsanalysis (existential approach to psychoanalysis), existential therapy, somatic psychotherapy, and the history and philosophy of medicine. Today more than ever there is an urgent need to recall, conserve, and evolve new approaches to medicine—approaches that still find absolutely no place in institutionalized medical research, training, and practice and are therefore at greater risk than ever before of falling into total historical oblivion—just when they are most called for.

MEDICAL ETHICS DEFINED

Medical ethics is a system of moral principles that applies values to the practice of clinical medicine and to scientific research. They are based on a set of values that professionals can refer to in the event that they are in conflict or are confused. The values include beneficence, nonmaleficence, and respect for autonomy (AMA, n.d.).

The AMA (n.d.) notes that the code of ethics is based on the understanding of the goals of medicine dating back to the fifth century BC and Hippocrates, the famous Greek physician. By 1847, the medical code of ethics was based greatly on Thomas Percival's work. He was an English physician-philosopher who wrote a code of medical ethics for hospitals in 1803 (AMA, n.d.).

Is Hippocrates important in the discussion of the meaning of meaning and the meaning of medical ethics? Yes, he is because that is where the drive to make the public understand that medicine was based on science and not on magical or religious activities that were used so often (Peel, 2005). Even so, those writings were put away and were not rediscovered until the Renaissance period in the early sixteenth century.

It was John Gregory, a professor of practice of physic in Edinburgh who published his lectures in which he redefined medical humanism in the context of the Scottish Enlightenment of philosophers such as David Hume (Peel, 2005). These letters opposed the work of Hobbes and his *Leviathan*. Gregory, like Hippocrates, wanted to set medicine apart and argued that medicine incorporated the ideal that physicians were empathetic and their practice was based on medical science (Peel, 2005).

The code is a living document, which means that it grows and evolves as new information is gained. The first edition came about in 1847. It did not change very much until 1903 when the language was updated. It was retitled *Principles of Medical Ethics (Principles)* (AMA, n.d.). It was again updated in 1949 and again in 1957. Minor changes were made in 1980. The 1957 version adopted a preamble along with ten statements of core values and commitments. The Judicial Council was given the authority of interpreting the ethical principles (AMA, n.d.).

According to many, including the AMA, the medical code of ethics has become too large.

The Code has become unwieldy—guidance on individual topics was hard to find; opinions varied significantly as to whether they offered general guidance or highly prescriptive statements. The interpretations were offered as the opinions of the Council on Ethical and Judicial Affairs (CEJA), which replaced the Judicial Council.

This writer can attest to the veracity of the previous statement. Just look at the "AMA Principles of Medical Ethics" (https://www.ama-assn.org/delivering-care/ama-principles-medical-ethics). Additionally, there are pages and pages throughout the internet from the AMA and other authors. They are worse than being unwieldy.

✿ Meaning of Meaning

How can this idea be defined? Seth Fontane Pennock (2016), cofounder of the Positive Psychology Program, said this:

> The question of meaning is not really one question but actually represents a cipher for a vast number of further questions. And

it is by no means obvious whether these questions are answerable at all; neither do we know with any certainty into which area of expertise the responsibility for answering these questions fall.

In fact, as this essay progresses, there will be a point where it is reported that many philosophers will not even touch this question. Instead, they push it on to spiritual or religious experts. That should tell us something about this search for meaning of meaning or what meaning means in medical ethics.

Even so, positive psychology has grappled with this question and continues work on attempting to define it. They begin with asking what meaning means in terms of the meaning of life.

✄ Medical Ethics Changes

Veatch (2006) argued that the philosophy of medicine changed medical ethics and traces thirty years to support his premise. Over the years, the core issues of philosophy included a stronger emergence of a more systematic and integrated thinking of the concept of medicine. During those years, biomedical ethics was introduced, and this brought about a change in thinking. In fact, the thoughts and opinions of bioethics changed dramatically over three decades.

The reshaping of these theories was most likely affected by the additional branches of ethics, such as those theories from Kant and his respect for people (Veatch, 2006). There is also the contribution that science made during decades, and this will continue to reshape ethics and philosophies in the next decades.

More than a decade ago, Duffy (2004) complained, "Modern medicine is currently confronting a crisis of meaning that is manifesting in a dispirited and demoralized profession" (p. 207). The search for meaning in medicine has been going on for decades. Duffy (2004) leaned on Socrates for support and affirmation for his ideas. It is in palliative care that Duffy (2004) believes meaning can be found because the most important factor in this field is compassion. This connects people to the Socratic ideal as well as rethinking the ethics of experience.

Duffy (2004) reported the stories of patients who taught him about meaning. A woman who had been strong was struck by cancer. She taught Duffy about the nature of suffering and that it is not about the disease; it is about the disconnection from things that were important to her. She withdrew from life and refused the help that all the people she had helped throughout her life. She taught Duffy that people create a metaphor so that there is a meaning to the experience. She found meaning there. She taught Duffy (2004) that healing is about being able to travel together along a journey to places that are most frightening to us. That healing is about the process to become whole through a transformation of ourselves to something that is complete in its own way (Duffy, 2004). The meaning of meaning is about the experience.

There was a man who was so sick and so depressed, and he died. He taught Duffy that healing is painful and frightening for both patient and doctor. The disease sucks up meaning from life, and the doctor or healer needs to be able to find that meaning and needs to construct a transformation for the patient. The healer must be able to find meaning for the patent and self and must be willing to travel through the dark places with the patient (Duffy, 2004).

The healer must be able to find meaning. Duffy did not learn it from books; he learned it from experiences. It is through these kinds of experiences that Duffy found wisdom. Duffy (2004) says he learned about the power of compassion through these learning experiences. He argued that it was compassion and the capacity of empathy that led to understanding meaning. To find meaning in their work, doctors need to experience the art of healing rather than falling back into the realm of scientific data. Further, as stated already, it is palliative medicine that can provide the philosophical foundation for a wisdom that is capable of including the power that the scientific method brings. This is the ethics of experience, according to Duffy (2004).

Given the fact that modern medicine is involved with HMOs and other groups telling doctors what they can and cannot do, there seems to be very little space for meaning given the focus on the bottom lines of those organizations. Duffy (2004) searched and searched but did not find his answers on meaning in his research. Instead, he found meaning in medicine through his interactions with patients who were dying. There, he was able to offer meaning through compassion.

Duffy (2004) related meaning to compassion. It was this wisdom he was searching for in his study. From some of his interviews and reading, he was led to believe that medical ethics was the key to wisdom. He researched things like justice, nonmalfeasance, autonomy, and beneficence, but as he said, all of that left him feeling safe but empty. He even found that the recent modern bioethics were nothing but a guide for managing anxious situations rather than the deeper meaning of his work as a physician. Duffy (2004) commented that these four were a well-constructed moral template, but they did not help him in his search for meaning. He clarified by saying that there is nothing wrong with these tenets; they just were not enough for him.

After discussing Hobbes, Socrates, and Galen, Duffy (2004) said that in recent times, even Zeus is stripped of his power and meaning because in the modern philosophers' thinking; the gods have been replaced by body parts. Of course, by modern science times, philosophers and others were using data and concluded that rational numbers and feelings were forgotten. He believes the world had become like Alice in Wonderland where everyone is a winner and gets a prize and said, "A philosophy that massacres meaning and leaves us each to fend for ourselves in a world where nothing stays the same" (Duffy, 2004, p. 210). This is not helpful.

Peel (2005) pointed out that contemporary bioethics is a collaboration of different experts, including philosophers of different theoretical schools. The deontologists tend to use a rule-based theory that follows along with Kant's work. The other major school in the discussion is the utilitarian, which follows along after the works of Bentham and measures and judges actions according to the consequences of the acts (Peel, 2005).

❈ Suspension of Meaning

Dell'Oro (2016) presented a metaphor provided by Warren Reich about meaning in medical ethics. While searching for meaning in medical ethics, Reich suggested that meaning might be illustrated by a stethoscope. Reich recounted that while a doctor was making rounds and checking vital signs, a patient asked him a question while he had his stereoscope on her chest, to which the doctor responded, "Quiet. I can't hear you while I'm listening" (Dell'Oro, 2016).

Dell'Oro (2016) explained that this metaphor is "emblematic of the inattention to meaning (not hearing) that was brought about by a reductionist focus in methodologies of modern scientific medicine and contemporary ethical theory" (Dell'Oro, 2016, p. 90).

Dell'Oro (2016) states that his essay has a commitment to the search for meaning. The author states that one of his major motivations is to encourage a dramatic shift in paradigms that focus on the interpretation of experiences. At the time of that writing, focus was on the experience of clinical practice with all of its inherent complexities. As the metaphor demonstrates, there is a mindset that has been created by modern scientific medicine.

Dell'Oro (2016) also argues that medicine cannot

be entirely equated with science because there are too many differences. For one thing, the primary goal of medicine is about bringing together actions that are both theoretical and practical simultaneously so that they will be good for the patient. He further concludes that given the modern mindsets regarding science and medicine, science eliminates the very questions of the meaning or meaninglessness of human existence (Dell'Oro, 2016). This is contrary to what clinical ethics should be promoting. These are the questions that medicine seems to suspend, which Dell'Oro, identifies as

> the significance of illness and disease, of our human condition as embodied, of birth, suffering and death, and of the service to the ethos of generosity that sustains the healing professions. (2016, p. 88)

❀ Overview/History of Medical Ethics

More than three decades ago, work that was deemed to be at the intersection of medicine and the humanities was typically referred to as "medical ethics." There was little discussion on the intersection of philosophy and medicine, but there was strong discussion that focused on clinical ethics. Integrating philosophy was seldom done. In fact, at that time, philosophy of medical ethics and philosophy of medicine were viewed as being completely separate fields. Medical ethics of that time emphasized moral topics that were often discussed in medical organizations or in religion. Philosophy of medicine emphasized conceptual and metaphysical issues that were divorced from medical ethics (Veatch, 2006).

In the 1970s, the historic field of medical ethics changed into an interdisciplinary field that involved experts and persons from an array of professions, such as lawyers, theologians, historians, social scientists, and of course, physicians and other health care professionals (Veatch, 2006).

The first major issue of discussion and debate was "informed consent," and for that, they brought in the ideas of Hippocrates and followers who were consequence-oriented professionals like Kant. (Consequences were mentioned a bit earlier.) They also brought in liberals, like Rousseau, Locke, Hobbes, and the Founding Fathers of the United States (Veatch, 2006).

Mental health was another big issue in medical ethics for this group in the 1970s. Physicians were being asked to do something such as certain surgeries that would control behavior. This involved removing or destroying parts of the brain believed to be fostering criminal behavior and violent behavior. Drugs were later introduced for children to control hyperactive behaviors (Veatch, 2006).

Philosophical work needed to happen to clarify these very controversial "treatments." They had to draw upon "the philosophy of mind, mind-body relations, and conceptual analysis of the notions of health and medicine" (Dell'Oro, 2016, p. 34). The work was focused on responsibility—on who was responsible.

Bioethicists attempted to seek a perspective that could sustain ethical discourse that attempted to address the value implication of technological developments in life sciences, in general, as well as in medicine, in particular. This perspective of meaning has a pluralistic character that encouraged anthropological interpretations in a theological manner. At the same time, the perspective was generally humanistic when it was not emphasizing nonreligious (Dell'Oro, 2016).

A major shift in medical ethics began toward the end of the 1970s. Medical ethics developed a preoccupation with the elaboration of normative criteria (so-called principles of respect of person, beneficence, nonmaleficence, and justice) that drew their justification from the perspective of a restrictive cluster of concepts in political philosophy (Dell'Oro, 2016, p. 87).

Peel (2005) also noted that the outcome of the deliberations on the early discussions of medical ethics led to an ethic that was based on those four principles: autonomy, justice, nonmaleficence, and beneficence. (These are mentioned throughout the essay because they are essential.) Nonmaleficence dates back to Hippocrates, and the ethic of not hurting people deliberately is the "cornerstone of rectifictory justice" (Peel, 2005, p. 172).

There was a push to develop a consensus among members that was apart from the horizon of meaning and meaningful narratives that initially aspired them. There was a strong influence to provide an ethical basis that was consistent for the public policy formation, moral philosophy that was developed for medical ethics an area of reflection that was centered on the use of rules and principles along with ethical theories that articulate them through the deontological or utilitarian approaches (Dell'Oro, 2016).

This perspective was criticized by Leon Kass regarding its inherent value or lack of value of having such principles because when these rules, etc. were applied to specific cases, they translated into doing good and not harm and to giving patients autonomy of decision-making, to promote and encourage equal access to health care, and to provide protection against biohazards. Dell'Oro (2016) reported further comments from Kass, whose conclusion was that

> as long as nobody is hurt, no one's will is violated, and no one is excluded or discriminated against, there is little to worry about. The possibility of willing dehumanization is out of sight and out of mind. (Dell'Oro, 2016, p. 89)

Dell'Oro (2016) goes on to say that the difficulty of moral reflection that addresses a number of questions about meaning is blamed on the complexity that exists with defining the "postmodern" condition. The modern scientific and philosophical agenda is known reason and optimism, so the definition of postmodernity must break through those ideas. There is also a structural fragmentation and contextual interpretation that defies any true image of totality. There is no clear philosophical theory regarding postmodernism as an accurate label in the area of philosophy.

As we pursue the meaning of meaning and the meaning of medical ethics, it is worthwhile to think about Viktor Frankl, a very famous Holocaust survivor. He was a Viennese doctor, psychiatrist, and neurologist who developed the logotherapy approach to therapy (Devoe, 2012). His theory was that anyone can get through almost anything if they have meaning in their life or if they have a purpose. The "central concept of logotherapy is meaning and the search for it in order to have the strength to surmount even the most difficult occurrences in life" (Frankl, 1962). His wife and family were killed; he knew it; he kept on fighting to follow a purpose in spite of his immense suffering. He believed one of man's primary goals is to discover the meaning of existence (Devoe, 2012).

Frankl (1962) realized that the prisoners who had something to hang on to fared better than those who just dwelt with the question of when they would get out of prison. People who could grab onto something had better mental health and thus better physical health. He said that even in a concentration camp, people had some opportunities to make decisions and to make choices, which provided them a sense of confidence and autonomy.

One of Frankl's (1962) first decisions had to do with a very precious manuscript he had written and which he had when he entered Auschwitz. Prisoners were told to leave everything in the room. He says he mentally extricated himself from his plans with the manuscript and other issues, and by this, Frankl was able to secure his psychological survival. In so doing, however, Frankl obliterated his life plan. Everything that could be taken from the prisoners was taken—psychologically, physically, emotionally.

He had one thing to hold onto. No matter what, the one thing nobody can take away is the ability to "choose one's attitude in any given set of circumstances, to choose one's own way" (Spriggs, 1998, p. 125).

Frankl was very strong in his theory that the will to meaning is a primary and universal human motivation (Wong, 2014). Sometimes, that motivation is not really conscious, but it is there. Fromm agreed and discussed the human's profound need for existential meaning. This was a unique theory in psychoanalysis and far from Freud's will for pleasure and the will for power as promoted by Adler and Nietzsche (Wong, 2014). Although Nietzsche did say, "He who has a *why* to live can bear almost any *how*" (Frankl, 1962).

✖ Can Meaning Be Retrieved

Dell'Oro (2016) argues that any attempt at moral reflection in the existentially charged realm of clinical ethics must begin with an open and free confrontation with the meaning of the experience (p. 91). Experience incorporates more than an empirical analysis that would lead to an etymological meaning. Experience brings in a reference to subjective intermediation. It is about a specific time and living through that time. It is about passing through a crisis and the growth an individual would achieve through this living. It leads to a response to the situation of crisis that holds meaning. This kind of crisis brings with it the need for reciprocity through the response that involves value. Dell'Oro (2016) asserts this leads to the idea of conscience.

Many clinicians involved in the debate have said that "questions of meaning" cannot be the priority; these questions can only have secondary importance in moments of crisis when tough decisions must be made (Dell'Oro, 2016). This, of course, makes sense. If a doctor hears a scream for help where survival is in question, the most important thing to do is to respond. Medical ethics are not going to be considered in such traumatic situations.

At other times, it makes sense to think about the meaning of medical ethics, but even then, there should be more thinking. Instead, most members of the profession are likely to think about clinical ethics in some sort of algorithm when facing a problem that must be solved. The author brings into the discussion the vast array of forms and rules that must be followed. Typically, the physicians use all these things as obstacles to steady, stable, and good decision-making. The problem is that very little can be solved or resolved by following a list of rules.

Citing Richard Zaner, Dell'Oro, (2016) commented that the person needs to be very alert in a number of ways to how the participants in the situation interrelate and the many diverse experiences they have and how they interpret these for self and others. In these situations, Dell'Oro (2016) says that the ethicist's involvement becomes a "work of circumstantial understanding" (p. 93).

Moral reasoning becomes especially important when questions of meaning need to be determined, as when those questions go beyond the implementation of normative strategies for solving these moral problems (Dell'Oro, 2016). Using this approach takes the problem-solver beyond "larger questions of meaning, questions for which ethicists have long declared their incompetence" (Dell'Oro, 2016, p. 98). At this point, ethicists pass on those questions to other venues, such as spiritual care persons, psychologists, or other agencies. Even so, clinical ethics continually attempt to answer these "meaning" questions. Since clinical ethicists continue to attempt to answer the meaning questions, clinical ethicists become more knowledgeable and better prepared to open the doors to many ideological confusions. In this process, these ethicists must be able to go past many ideological prejudices that are already embedded in the archeology of meaning.

Dell'Oro (2016) argues that today's medical people face an enormous stereotype that they can fix anything. That is simply not true. Physicians—in fact, all people—need to understand that when curing is not possible, they need to have "an appreciation for the deepest matters of our humanity" (Dell'Oro, 2016, p. 98). They need to understand that curing may not be possible but caring continues to be possible. This is where meaning comes into active play in that the meaning of care changes. It does so mostly in times of vulnerability where nothing more can be done (Dell'Oro, 2016).

Clinical ethics must view medicine as a human practice. Clinical ethics must also act as a reminder of the ultimate nature of ethics in medicine. It is an interpretation of moral experiences and moral norms.

❊ What Would Happen if Medical Ethical Codes Were Eliminated?

We know from mass communication sources that countless medical errors are made every day. Johns Hopkins (2016) reported that medical errors were now the third leading cause of death in the United States. More than 250,000 deaths each year are due to medical errors. The CDC reports thousands fewer, but Johns Hopkins reports that the CDC does not classify medical errors separately on death certificates. This skews the count.

People should not conclude that all those doctors and health care personnel were bad. Still, this number is absurdly high and needs to be brought down to zero. If there were no code of ethics at all, there would be a lot more medical errors and wrong decisions made. Consider some of the principles of medical ethics.

Duffy (2014) said that ethics are necessary; they are critical in order to save man from himself. According to Hobbes's philosophy, man is always in a constant struggle between his animal nature and his higher moral sense. The only way to control these struggles, according to Hobbes, is to construct social systems that will rein in man so that nurture wins over nature. Darwin's theories seem to support at least some of Hobbes's thoughts with the primary theory of the fittest being the survivors.

These ideas can be seen in some of the works of Huxley, Dawkins, and other philosophers and scientists who argue that ethics must not be established or founded on human nature because there is an "[unbridgeable gap between the selfishness of our natural inclinations and the necessary selfishness of our moral duties" (Duffy, 2004, p. 209). In other words, human intuition cannot be trusted. This means that it is not what people experience but what people construct in their minds that matters.

Here is the statement from Duffy: we cannot go backward to the theories and ethics of the past; we must move forward. Darwin was certainly correct about evolution. It continues no matter what any of us do. Duffy said, "Any philosophy must be capable of embracing this change" (p. 210). Schlegel and Hegel said the same thing: there is not going back; there is no return to nature. Duffy (2004) suggests that the answer for finding meaning and for constructing an ethical code is dependent upon combining the Romantics' prerational approach with the Enlightenment schools' rational materialism. It was strongly recommended, and it sounds good, but like all philosophies, a strong voice in the future or a change in technology and society's thoughts of morals changes anything quickly.

The question that must remain in the forefront is this: can this theory or these theories help the profession to understand what meaning means and will it lead to meaning in the ethical code?

These stories lead to a conclusion that is it important to

understand the meaning in medicine. They also indirectly promote having a strong code of medical ethics, a code that has meaning to everyone.

If there were a suspension of meaning of medical ethics, the outcomes would be really negative. We already know that there are more people of all ages harmed through medical care, including in hospitals and other facilities. Ethical codes require health care providers to report errors and to report all facts about the patient.

The AMA Principles of Medical Ethics is comprised of a preamble and nine principles (AMA, 2018). Principle II says that "physicians need to strive to report physicians deficient in character or competence, or engaging in fraud or deception, to appropriate entities" (AMA, 2018). How many physicians do not report observations they have made that led them to believe that another doctor was incompetent or misled the patient? This writer suspects that many physicians do not follow this principle. Certainly, some do, but consider how many medical errors result in death each year—at least 250,000.

Principle VIII says that a physician "shall, while caring for a patient, regard responsibility to the patient as paramount" (AMA, 2018). This writer knows of a physician who refused to complete a health form that a patient needed for another issue. This is not helping the patient because it caused the patient months of anxiety. (He eventually completed it.)

Principles VI and IX are slightly contradictory. Principle VI says the physician can choose the people he will serve (AMA, 2018), which seems very reasonable. Principle IX says the physician shall support access to medical care for all people. This needs to be researched because it seems that a physician, like any other businessperson or service person, should be able to refuse service to whomever he or she wants, but then it seems to say the physician must support access to all.

Frankl also said that ethics were crucial for life. Wong and Reilly (2017) say that Frankl's self-transcendence model is practical because it came about from struggling with the "ethical challenges of how to be a decent human being" while under negative conditions in life: living with a sense of dignity and importance in this life even as people face massive abuse, death, and degradation and how to prevent people in power from becoming monsters like so many well-known devils.

Frankl's response was to awaken the will to meaning to search for one's self-transcendence; to practice the meaning mindset in order to find the truth, beauty, and goodness in all situations one faces in life; and to develop and cultivate personal responsibility to do the right thing in all those situations (Wong and Reilly, 2017). These things will lead to a good life that is calm and stable, and if one has a stable mental and emotional life, one will also have a good physical life.

These three tactics need to be adopted by the medical profession as medical ethics. If all health care professional adopted and engaged in those three activities, there would hardly need to be a code of medical ethics because those in the profession would already be acting ethically in every situation. Wong and Reilly (2017) said, "Frankl's model provides a practical framework to live a virtuous life of ST [self-transcendence] with a philosophical foundation in virtue ethics." This may be the place to begin to retrieve medical ethics in a more useful format.

CHAPTER 1
INTRODUCTION

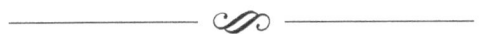

Anticipation shows itself as the possibility of understanding one's own most and extreme potentiality-of-being, that is, as the possibility of authentic existence. Its ontological constitution must be made visible by setting forth the concrete structure of anticipation of death.

—Martin Heidegger, *Being and Time*

❀ Background

MARTIN HEIDEGGER RECOGNIZED ONE OF THE foundational elements in relation to man's progression through the life span: individuals continually seek self-understanding and authenticity of existence as they move toward death (246). As people move toward the end of the life span, they may face issues related to unachieved goals or potential that result in the onset of anxiety or fear of death. Creating support mechanisms for individuals during this time requires a close scrutiny of psychotherapeutic approaches and theories that relate to self-awareness, the meaning or purpose of existence, the role of fear, anxiety, and guilt, and the implications for individual psychosocial functioning.

In the development of a psychoanalytic approach for elderly populations, it is essential to understand the foundations of psychotherapy and the implications for those facing death. During this time, people attempt to bring together their understanding of the meaning of existence and frequently respond with anxiety and fear. The existential orientation in psychotherapeutic paradigms is related directly to the sense of a connection between experience and psychological functioning (May and Yalom 1). Major theorists supporting existential psychotherapy emerged in the mid-20th century and included Freud, Jung, Frankl, Maslow, Erickson, May, Husserl, and Rogers. These existential therapists believed that experiences of fear, anxiety, and guilt can take on different forms, including both normal and neurotic forms that can be assessed within a therapeutic experience.

Within the parameters of a psychotherapeutic praxis, there are four constitutive concerns that become pivotal in end-of-life experiences: isolation, meaninglessness, freedom, and death. Confrontational experiences related to these axiomatic elements become the foundation for existential exploration within a therapeutic paradigm. For elderly individuals, the interplay among these elements can also become a focus of psychological responses, including the development of anxiety responses. In addressing anxiety, fear, and end-of-life experiences, an existential and interpretive direction can be applied to the creation of a psychotherapeutic praxis. In developing this type of approach, it is essential to understand the nature of the problem, relate the issue of death to philosophically derived perspectives, and shape an interpretive assessment of existing paradigms.

✕ Nature of the Problem

The creation of a new response to the psychotherapeutic needs of an aging population relates directly to the transformation of the modern culture and the shift in views on meaningfulness and authenticity in life as well as active decision-making during the process of dying and death. Modern social culture has been impacted by the transformation of views of death from a systematic component of the life cycle to an event to be avoided at all costs. This has led to the medicalization of death and the sequestering or sidelining of death. In essence, modern changes in medical technology and changing cultural views have led to the perception that death is an event that should be unequivocally avoided whenever possible. As a result of this view, dying can be prolonged, painful, and uncomfortable and can require the application of many different technological advances and medical approaches that influence how individuals perceive death.

Medical technologies have waylaid death and provided support for separating people from the discomfort and messiness of end-of-life care (Beach and Morrison 2057). Contemporary practical consciousness sanctions the sequestration of death and all its mess, disorder, pain, and trouble from public view. Individuals are thus protected from the need to feel pity and empathy in face-to-face encounters (though such sentiments may be expressed in a "staged" way if that is seen to be appropriate) (McKenzie 119).

Modern medicine has not only increased the number of people who are being cared for in institutional settings but has also changed the public attitudes about illness, dying, and death. While a century ago people were cared for primarily in their homes by loved ones, modern medicine has played a "solution-based" approach on the issue of dying, placing people in hospitals and health care institutions to address the "problem" of death. Loved ones no longer embrace the direct care experience of death with their family members, and the medicalization of death has led to methods to prevent it. Denial of the immediacy and inevitability of death have become a part of the modern culture.

Death and dying and the changing patterns of care have led to a cultural perspective that places negative stigmatization on illness and aging, both of which are natural factors that impact individuals throughout the life span. Because of the modern culture's denial of death, the impact from a social level is significant. People, communities, and even lawmakers have struggled with approaches to addressing the "problem" of death, including creating responses to chronic or terminal illnesses and the marginalization of the elderly.

Sequestration has emerged as a cultural and social response to the issue of aging, a growing aging population, and prolonged processes of dying and death. Sequestration theory provides a foundation for understanding the social changes that have occurred and the desire to deny and emancipate individuals from the experience of death. Willmott cited Anthony Giddens when assessing sequestration theory and presenting a view of how modernity has changed our views of dying and death. Giddens maintained that modern consumer culture has led to a "'purchasing' of ontological security through institutions and routines that protect us from direct contact with madness, criminality, sexuality, nature and death" (Willmott 649). Willmott further argued that this focus has resulted in a sequestration of experiences that are notably disquieting, especially experiences that are difficult or create inherent uneasiness. The unpredictability of death even in the presence of all the best efforts to make it predictable is one of the central factors that have led to the cultural rejection of the experience (Stanley and Wise 947).

The routines created to address the "problem" of death are linked to the desire to sequester the experience or to deny its force. Religious rituals that constantly remind participants of their mortality are created to address the emotional messiness of the experience. From a broader cultural perspective though, the use of different institutions, from hospitals to funeral homes, to create a structure for death provides some comfort even when death occurs unpredictably. These types of institutions focus on the institutions and their components and not on the actual process of dying or death and succeed in making death invisible. A person can go through a process of dying in an institution, be removed after death, be whisked away to a funeral home, be dressed up nicely and placed in a closed coffin, and be buried in the ground without the members of the family having to take any part in the difficult reality.

Though from a practical perspective, the ability to prevent troublesome or uneasy experiences may seem beneficial, there are theorists who believe that this approach has led to a variety of other problems, including the lack of an understanding of the value that death has and the importance of death as a social experience, and the importance of addressing the needs of the dying as a component of the living. The sanitization of death diminishes its relevance as a part of life and results in the denial of mortality. Willmott also cited the work of Mellor and Shilling (423) in developing an understanding of this process, because they reflected on the need to maintain a transpersonal and existential focus on death and to recognize its significance as both a part of the social discourse and in relation to individual experiences. The lack of knowledge and acceptance of death (or the denial of death) can inherently impact the way in which people value life.

Rich, in a January 2007 article entitled "Causation and Intent: Persistent Conundrums in End-of-Life Care," reflected upon the conflicting views that relate to a culture that has lost the experience of dying and death, specifically the rejection of end-of-life experiences that allow elderly people to process the progression toward death. This has led to debates about the nature of methods that are used to end life, methods to ensure that dying and death can be compartmentalized, and methods to ensure that death is a clean and acceptable process.

One of the central problems in the sequestration of death and the increasing use of institutional methods of securing a tidy death is that people pay closer attention to the legal parameters set by the government than the actual reality of death itself. Individuals may have a very distinct view on how life is defined (e.g., the right to life movement has made distinct statements about when life begins), but dying and death are much less easily defined concepts. In truth, everyone is dying from the time they are born. The inevitability of death is one of the most frightening aspects of human existence. Correspondingly, individuals deny death—deny its immediacy, even at the point when death is impending. The use of medical technologies to relinquish control over the process and to prolong life in denial of death has become one of the costliest components of modern society. Measures to ensure that life is prolonged regardless of the costs have led to a cultural message fostering fear and denial of authentic experiences at the end of life.

The sequestering of death, including the identification of death as a "problem" to be solved, has increased psychological manifestations of anxiety and conflict in elderly population. The cultural shift in views of death and the medicalization of the problem of death have led to high levels of death anxiety, a lack of a dialogue about the authentic experiences of death, and a lack of belief that a coherent sequence of life is valuable to human experience.

✣ Purpose of the Study

The purpose of this study is to explore an existential psychoanalytical framework that can be applied to addressing the needs of elderly populations to create an authentic experience and address anxiety and "death fear" within a social culture rejecting the value of the experience of death. The creation of an existential praxis that can support the presence of anxiety while also addressing the personal manifestations of anxiety has been noted by theorists including May. The therapist's role, May maintained, was to address the issue of anxiety and fear that can prevent a person from experiencing life and confronting death while not alleviating anxiety altogether. May argued that life cannot be fully lived or death fully addressed without the conflict that emerges as a result of anxiety. Creating a response to individual needs that reduces anxiety to "tolerable levels" can be a construct of an existential psychotherapeutic praxis.

Experiential psychoanalytical views reflect a clear distinction between anxiety and fear and relate a function for each. Anxiety occurs in many different types of situations and is a response to the threat to personal autonomy and the need for survival. The creation for conflict that is based on an innate survival instinct is not an issue to be resolved as a part of the therapeutic process. Anxiety itself is not inherently bad. May maintained that anxiety is a "threat to our existence or to values we identify in our existence." The processing of anxiety within an existential psychoanalytical praxis can support greater self-awareness, reduce physical manifestations of anxiety, and prevent debilitating responses to anxiety.

Anxiety and fear are distinctly connected, and an assessment of the role of death fear in addressing the needs of elderly populations is a significant consideration. Fear is another natural process that results in the presence of a threat to autonomy, physical safety, or life. Fear is a much more rationalized process and reflects a set of beliefs about the conditions an individual experiences and the progression of those experiences as a part of the natural life span. Anxiety is a much baser response to the presence of fear and reflects physiological and psychological response components that can influence an individual's capacity for functioning.

The purpose of this study is to identify an existential psychoanalytical praxis that can be used with elderly patients, especially those experiencing anxiety and death fear as they progress through the life span. This approach includes an evaluation of the different elements impacting psychological and psychosocial functioning, including the physiological, psychological, social, and spiritual factors that influence adjustment to aging.

❈ Definitions

Anxiety: Anxiety is a set of physiological and psychological responses to the presence of "personal need to survive, to preserve our being, and to assert our being" (May and Yalom 3). Normal anxiety is in proportion to the situation, does not result in repression, and can be used to address a dilemma that might be anxiety provoking. Anxiety responses can include increased heart rate, increased blood pressure, and a sense of apprehension, but they can also include debilitating or destructive choices.

Neurotic anxiety is not appropriate to the situation, is frequently repressed, and does not support constructive conflict that can alleviate the situation from which the anxiety arose.

Autonomy: Autonomy reflects the right of the client/patient to personal decision-making. Autonomy requires supporting the process that needs to occur to ensure that a person has the greatest level of self-determination possible.

Beneficence: Beneficence is the responsibility of the therapist to contribute to the welfare of the patient. Beneficence is the process of promoting well-being and ensuring that the most appropriate level of care is provided. Achieving a level of well-being for the client/patient may include everything from therapeutic interventions with the aim of improved psychological and physical functioning to support for the process of dying and death. Beneficence suggests a goal of the achievement of wellness but does not preclude the notion that care can support well-being during natural human processes, including those that result in the end of life (Curran 1; Tauber 3).

Death fear: Death fear is a morbid, abnormal, and persistent fear of death that inhibits authentic participation in experiences of life (Collett and Lester 179).

Existential psychoanalysis: A psychotherapeutic

approach that supports patient exploration of experiences and meaning. Inherent in the existential psychotherapeutic approach is the belief that conflict is beneficial in responding to fundamental questions of existence and relating these to anxiety and death fear.

❊ Research Questions

The following questions were used to guide assessments of the feasibility and implementation of an existential psychoanalytic praxis for use with elderly patients. The results of this research were expected to offer insight into the physical, mental, social, and spiritual elements impacting psychological functioning in response to anxiety and death fear.

Q1. The first research question was addressed through the integration of qualitative data collected from participating therapists. The research question is this: How feasible is the application of the proposed existential psychoanalytic praxis to the process of care for elderly patients?

Q2. The second research question was the basis for the quantitative segment of the research study. This question is this: After implementing the newly designed existential psychoanalytic praxis for a period of five weeks, how effective is the approach in meeting the needs of elderly clients/patients? Specifically, will these individuals demonstrate improvements in regard to their specific individual goals, reductions in anxiety responses, and reductions in death fear?

Q3. The last question allowed for the integration of qualitative data collected from patients. How successfully were the therapists at implementing the existential psychoanalytic praxis, and how successful was the praxis in improving self-awareness and reducing anxiety?

❊ Significance of the Problem

The aging of the American population has led to a significant challenge in meeting the needs of a large population over the age of sixty-five. In 2009, people over the age of sixty-five comprised 12.9 percent of the US population, or 39.6 million Americans (Administration on Aging 1). Projections by the Administration on Aging suggest that by 2030, there will be about 72.1 million elderly people in the United States, more than twice the number in 2000 (1). The Centers for Disease Control and Prevention (CDC) estimate that about 20 percent of the population over the age of fifty-five currently experiences some form of mental health issue (2). Anxiety is noted as the most significant mental health concern, followed by cognitive impairment and mood disorders like depression. Suicide rates among elderly Americans is especially high, with men over the age of eighty-five taking their own lives at a rate of about 45.23 per 100,000 as compared to an overall rate of 11.01 per 100,000 for all ages (CDC 2).

Mental distress, or the presence of symptoms associated with anxiety and/or depression, is a problem in elderly populations. Mental distress can have a negative impact on the ability of elderly individuals to participate in activities of daily living, maintaining their homes, working, or sustaining interpersonal relationships (CDC 5). Almost 10 percent of the elderly population indicates some level of mental distress that impacts their capacity for functioning (CDC 5). One of the challenges identified by the CDC in their study of mental health issues in the elderly is that anxiety is prevalent but may be underreported because many people believe that anxiety and death fear that detracts from activities and life experiences is a normative part of the progression of aging (CDC 8). The presence of anxiety and lack of social support mechanisms are significant contributory factors to loss of quality of life in elderly populations (Strine et al. 151).

The problem of addressing the psychological and psychosocial responses to end-of-life experiences relates directly to the urgency of death as a "boundary situation" that propels individuals into an assessment of life meaning. As individuals confront death, they are faced with questions about the nature of their lives and the implications for determining the value of life. Some of the questions that may have seemed less urgent at other times in life become essential to the reality of the aging process. An individual able to postpone discussion of life purpose can see the parameters of life and the need for immediacy in their experiences. Subsequently, elderly individuals may explore a greater level of self-understanding and require the application of existential therapeutic perspectives to garner some understanding of purpose and experience. Because death fear and anxiety can have a very real impact on the capacity of people to participate in their lives as they age, this study provides an important reflective assessment of an approach that can help to moderate for neurotic psychological responses.

✻ Assumptions and Limitations

This study was based on the assumption that therapists or practitioners working with elderly patients could apply an existential psychoanalytical approach based on the praxis developed. Further, the study is also based on the adequacy of data collected from existing studies that indicate the significant of anxiety and death fear as factors influencing elderly populations and the value perceived in applying a therapeutic process to addressing these issues. This study is also linked to the assumption that participants in this kind of psychoanalytical process will demonstrate a willingness to participate reflectively and share information regarding their levels of participation with candor.

This study is limited by a focus on a single existential psychoanalytical paradigm that is identified, rather than a comparison of multiple approaches. This study is also limited by regionality, based on the need for an assessment of the application of the praxis in clinical settings and conducting interviews with practitioners applying this strategic approach to the care of elderly clients/patients.

❊ Ethical Assurances

The ethics of this research study were defined in relation to the research application, approval process, and the information provided to the subjects before participation. The study was designed to be fully compliant with *The Belmont Report*. *The Belmont Report* has remained a significant ethical reference point for many Institutional

Review Boards (Schrag 494). The current study was described and detailed fully in a formal Institutional Review Board (IRB) application and was approved before any data were collected about practitioners or patients.

The Belmont Report of 1979 outlined three fundamental ethical principles which should be applied when undertaking any research on human subjects: respect for individuals, beneficence, and justice. Researchers are required to maintain respect for the individuals, protect autonomy, treat those involved in research with courtesy, and ensure that there is informed consent. Researchers are required to be truthful, without the presence of any deception. Researchers are required to incorporate the essence of beneficence, the concept of "doing no harm," with research undertaken in a manner that will minimize any risks while maximizing potential benefit. Finally, researchers are required to consider justice, which refers to the way that research should be designed so that it is not exploitative, so that it is reasonable and has a fair distribution of the costs and benefits across all participants. All three requirements were adhered to during the design and implementation of this study.

A particular challenge with this research was the vulnerable nature of the sample population to be used in the study; not only were some of the participants elderly, but some members of the sample group may also have had impaired cognitive abilities. Other less vulnerable subjects could not have been used to learn about the impact of the existential therapeutic praxis on outcomes related to mediation for anxiety and death fear.

The research design satisfied the three main ethical criteria, with particular consideration of the vulnerable nature of the population. Informed consent, in writing, was gained from the patients or assigned guardians of the potential sample, following a briefing on the purpose and the nature of the study. The patients/guardians of subjects were provided with an informed consent document, which identified the process of the study, the purpose, and the necessary protective measures for each subject. In addition, permission to observe, record, and note anecdotal data was requested from both the patient and therapists, who were also required to participate in the interviews.

❧ Summary

The process of aging brings with it questions of the meaning of existence, sense of self-worth, and social, spiritual, and psychological beliefs that can influence individual functioning. Anxiety and death fear increase in prevalence as individuals age and can be impacted by health issues, changes in psychological functioning, and loss of ability to participate fully in experience of daily living. Almost 10 percent of the elderly population in the United States has experienced some level of anxiety, depression, or death fear that impacts their capacity for participation in the activities of daily living.

Though many different therapeutic approaches have been applied to the treatment of elderly individuals, current approaches do not address all of the elements impacting the functions of individuals in later stages of the life span. An interpretive existential praxis can be utilized to determine successes in the treatment of older individuals and can promote a sense of well-being while also maintaining conflict necessary to ensure continued participation in life.

This research study was designed to assess the range of different schools of thought that influence the development of a psychoanalytical praxis built on existential principles. The central premise behind this study is that the application of an existential psychotherapeutic approach that will address both anxiety and death fear in aging adults and promote an analytical process by which self-awareness and personal exploration can occur. This results in the creation of an operational psychoanalytic model that addresses the issue of the fear of death and the subsequent anxiety that can occur from unresolved issues surrounding the anticipation of death. This research study is designed to assess the models or psychoanalytical praxes introduced when addressing the needs of elderly individuals and evaluate both the historical context in which they were formed and the support mechanisms for their continuation. Through a close scrutiny of existing approaches, the evidence presented supports the benefits of existential and pathosophical praxis to create responsive options for elderly patients seeking support at the end of life.

CHAPTER 2
ANALYTICAL REVIEW
OF LITERATURE

THE CONCEPT OF APPLYING AN EXISTENTIAL perspective to a psychoanalytic praxis has a historical foundation in existential psychological and existential psychotherapy. Irving Yalom explored the creation of an existential psychotherapeutic approach by relating a number of views of the progression of existential philosophical principles, maintaining that many leading therapists have applied existential principles in therapy (5). Yalom also maintained that many early influential psychologists, including Wilhelm Wundt, Sigmund Freud, Edward Titchner, Carl Rogers, and Gordon Allport, used existential elements in their exploration of the roots of psychopathology. Correspondingly though, the existential components of the work of many of these theorists represent more of a "subtle accent" that these therapists "unwittingly employ," rather than praxis utilized for the substantive purpose of psychoanalysis.

This view of the implicit perspective of psychologists toward the application of existentialism may be the underlying reason that many therapists supported a shift away from existential questioning toward more overt behavioral elements. Essentially, the existential questions that drove the therapeutic process appeared too vague and without clear connections between the principles and the central angst of those seeking therapy. The previous existential approaches were viewed in some regard as imprecise and muddled, suggesting that existential psychology was not actually based on a specific method that could be described as a science of the mind (Merleau-Ponty 382). The move toward a more scientific approach to psychology led to the perception that an existential paradigm could not meet the rigors of scientific exploration.

Over the past thirty years, the pendulum has swung, with theorists recognizing the significance of assessing the range of influences of existential exploration on psychological functioning, psychopathology, and the psychotherapeutic process. Growth of the field of experimental existential psychology has brought into alignment new views on some traditional theorists.

Reflecting on the principles and research of leading theorists who have applied existential principles, including Freud, Jung, Maslow, Erickson, May, Yalom, Husserl, and Rogers, it is possible to apply existential questioning to the exploration and analytical assessment of psychological functioning. Research into the views of these psychologists provides a foundation for creating an existential psychoanalytic praxis to be applied in therapeutic relationships with elderly populations facing the end of life.

❌ Background

One of the struggles in developing a comprehensive assessment of the background of existentialism is that there are foundations in a number of traditions, including philosophy, psychology, and psychiatry. William Barrett outlined some central principles regarding the application of the term "existentialism," maintaining that it begins with a philosophical view of man's struggle to understand essential questions about the "human condition in its totality" (126). Barrett maintained that existence precedes essence, so man's understanding of the purposeful nature of existence was essential to relating man's essential capabilities.

Man exists and makes himself what he is; his individual essence or nature comes out of his existence, and in this sense, it is proper to say that existence precedes essence. Man does not have a fixed essence that is handed to him ready-made; rather, he makes his own nature out of his freedom and the historical conditions in which he is placed (Barrett 102).

In alignment with this view, the progression of questions about life, purpose, meaning, and death all become significant in defining a rationale for existence. Barrett believed that this was a component of the uniqueness of the human condition because man seeks answers to questions that seem either essentially simplistic or seemingly unanswerable. Rollo May maintained that existentialism did not represent a single school of thought or area of exploration in philosophy or psychology but "an attitude, an approach to human beings, rather than a special school or group" (185). May's perspective was linked to the identification of existentialism as a foundational view that could be applied to an analytical science in which the human condition or human identity is explored.

The modern connection between existentialism and psychoanalysis began in the post-World War II era, when existentialism emerged as a method of exploring states of mind and applied the views of Kierkegaard, Nietzsche, Heidegger, and Sartre by a group of psychologists and psychiatrists, including Ludwig Binswanger, Viktor Frankl, and many others (Feist and Feist 341). These Europeans focused on the application of scientific study but also incorporated an assessment of some of the broader questions and sought methods to scrutinize the progression of the human psyche. In the United States, theorists like psychologist Rollo May and psychiatrist Irving Yallom applied an existential perspective to exploring the experiential expressions of essential questioning and the implications of conflict for the progression of the psychological states. In understanding the foundations of existential psychology and psychiatry, it is valuable to understand the foundations in European existentialism and the application of theoretical principles that drove a movement more than a half century ago.

Martin Heidegger

Though existentialism as a concept goes back to the authorship of nineteenth-century philosophers, including Friedrich Schelling, Soren Kierkegaard, Franz Kafka, and Friedrich Nietzsche, Martin Heidegger's evaluation of the philosophical principles of existentialism have been applied to the development of a science of the mind constructed around the concept of man's essential questioning. Heidegger (1889–1976) was born in Messkirch, Germany, and was influenced as a student by the writings of Kierkegaard and Nietzsche, as well as the mentorship of Edmund Husserl (Krell 5). Heidegger identified the significance of exploring essential questions of existence but reflected on the contextual nature of human experience and the correlation between experiential and temporal components.

Heidegger's philosophical principles regarding the nature of human experience and the analytical views of how man self-assesses in the presence of specific conditions become elements of a psychological existential process. Heidegger maintained that man continually tries to understand the purpose or meaning of existence within the scope of man's experiences in a temporal world. Heidegger described his views of being, or in his case "Dasein," as a central entity in direct contrast with "nonexistence." Because of the purposeful nature of existence and the belief in man's capacity, Dasein is constantly driven by the question of wholeness and approaches that help to determine both potential and meaning within man's experiential perspective (Heidegger 280). "As long as Dasein is as an entity, it has reached its 'wholeness'" (Heidegger 280). Subsequently, man is driven by to continually create and recreate a sense of true self and to apply an authentic and experiential view of self within the world.

Heidegger's views are especially important when considering the nature of man's development within a world and his belief in the temporality of experience or the immediacy of the need for answers to central questions. Man seeks a greater understanding of his existence in a specific environment and the meaning of existence, as well as the meaning of nonexistence. "Within the horizon of time the projection of a meaning of 'Being' in general can be accomplished." More completely, it is plausible to maintain that existential conundrums emerge from a very real assessment that Dasein exists temporally and that man's time on earth, or within any conscious existence, will someday end. As man explores his understanding of being in time, he must also recognize the significance of exploring a closer understanding of being toward death.

Heidegger also recognized that existential exploration and the seeking of answers to fundamental questions of purpose and meaning frequently occurred in relation to dramatic events or the progression toward death. Individuals consciously explore existential concerns when pervasive factors, including the aging, provide an impetus or a temporal directive for scrutinizing life experiences. Subsequently, Heidegger's existentialism stood as a foundation for understanding the contextual nature of experience and the importance of defining influencing factors that support answer-seeking behaviors.

❈ Jean Paul Sartre

Jean Paul Sartre (1905–1980) identified some elements of existentialism that can be applied both in the creation of a definition that can be applied to psychoanalytical processes and in defining elements to be included in a psychoanalytical praxis. Meaningfulness for many of the philosophers of the nineteenth century was related directly to the significance of God and of defining the existence of God. Contrary to this position, Sartre explored Heidegger's contextualized perspective on man's existence absent of the application of God. Sartre, a French-born atheist, explored the essential questions of meaning and being by recognizing that an essentially struggles with issues of alienation. It was Sartre's contention that existential therapeutic approaches had to seek to bridge the gap between the angst-creating empirical issues that man faced and the "original model in which each man has chosen his being" (115).

Sartre shared a view of the importance of a contextualized being (being in world) with Heidegger and believed that some of the struggles that man experiences on a psychological level extend from a sense of disconnection between truth and meaning. Subsequently, Sartre developed a phenomenological approach to analyzing the exploration of individual understanding. Sartre supported the value of an existential phenomenology for psychoanalysis, supporting the deconstruction of modern hermeneutics and creating a systematic approach to addressing man's response to what occurs in the world. Both Sartre and Heidegger maintained the contextualized nature of man's experiences. In relating the creation of an existential phenomenology, Sartre set the foundation for studies of man's experiences, history, and social context as they influenced psychological functioning. This provided a foundation for the exploration of existentialism as a premise for psychoanalytical processes introduced by Freud, Binswanger, Jung, Erikson, and Rogers.

✂ Freud

German psychologist Sigmund Freud (1856–1939) contextualized the development of self, providing support for existentialism as a means of understanding the progression of psychopathology. Freud looked at the early formation of relational interactions and the development of relationships as a means of determining man's sense of self in the world (Freud and Strachey 41). Relational attributes of trust between mother and child have a lasting impact on relationships that form through life. Lack of trust attributed to a lack of maternal attention in infancy, for example, can play a role in the conflicts and trust expressed in relationships later in life. Freud explored the nature of repressed emotions or beliefs, the nature of compulsions, and the implications for determining existence over essence (Freud 145).

It was Freud's contention that a psychoanalytical process had to reflect an understanding of the role of contextual factors that led to the progression of the psyche. Freud believed the uncovering unconscious influencing forces that determine the progression of compulsions can be the purpose of a therapeutic process (Freud 145–146).

Freud recognized that the progression of the psyche through developmental stages ultimately led to the ability of the individuals to demonstrate balance between essential conflicts, like sexual urges and personal control. Adulthood as a developmental stage was reflective of the ability of adults to create balance between different aspects of life through the application of restraint. This related to the ability attributable to the ego, of repressing or controlling unconscious thoughts and control of behavioral impulses. While this placed a context around the experiential components of man's existence, it did not drive the exploration of specific concepts or a broader exploration of existential angst.

Freud did relate the conflict that man feels in attempting to balance elements of experience and larger questions of purpose of worth. Happiness is a concept that is often related to a range of different stages of psychosocial development and sometimes misidentified with satisfaction in regard to Freud. Sexual satisfaction or gratification and happiness are clearly two different elements in relation to psychosocial development. Freud related happiness in terms of the ability to create balance between physical demands and intellectual or emotional development. Subsequently, this kind of balance was achieved through a push and pull between manifestation of power and the ability to repress behaviors. Freud's assessment of repression, the unconscious mind, and foundational views on man's essential angst have been linked to the assessment of existential purpose and the ability of individuals to derive meaning from action.

❇ Binswanger and Frankl

The early existential psychologists and psychiatrists emerged in Europe and were linked to the influences of philosophers like Heidegger, Sartre, and Edmund Husserl as well as the psychoanalytic views of Freud. Swiss-born psychologist Ludwig Binswanger (1881–1966) recognized the value of Freud's views on the mind but also sought a greater connection to the philosophical principles of Kierkegaard and Heidegger related to man's notion of self in the world.

Binswanger's perspective clearly supported the application of an existential perspective and the integration of this perspective in relating functional views of psychological functioning.

> It is a question of attempting to understand and to explain the human being in the totality of his/her existence. But that is possible only from the perspective of our total existence: in other words, only when we reflect on and articulate our total existence, the "essense" and "form" of being human. (Frie 22–23)

From this perspective, Binswanger built on Heidegger's Dasein and applied methods to assess the nature of being in the world and being beyond the world. The potentiality of Binswanger's conceptual view of being provided a basis from which psychoanalytical processes could be expounded.

Austrian psychiatrist Viktor Frankl's (1905–1997) humanistic psychology was linked to the views of Binswanger and Heidegger and defined by the premise of absolutes that were identified by authors like Irvin Yalom. Frankl's experiences though defined a much more concrete application of existential perspectives through his work in the concentration camps of Nazi Germany. Frankl argued that any understanding of the human condition had to reflect the belief in the inevitability of death, existential isolation, and even the conflict that can arise from a sense of meaninglessness. In his concentration camp experiences, Frankl explored some of the central premises of human existence and sought insight into the truth of the human condition. It was Frankl's contention that "love is the ultimate and the highest goal to which Man can aspire" (Frankl 56). Like Freud's contention that each step in human development was inextricably linked to past and innate responses to seemingly unconscious drives, Frankl believed that self-actualization and the realization of self-worth were shaped by value placed on love. "The salvation of Man is through love and in love. I understood how a man who has nothing left in this world still may know bliss, be it only for a brief moment, in the contemplation of his beloved" (Frankl 56).

❈ Rollo May

American existential psychologist Rollo May (1909–1994) is often associated with Frankl and theologian Paul Tillich in regard to his views on existentialism and its essential nature in determining what many saw as an evolution of the psychology of the mind (Feist and Feist 343). In the 1950s, May applied qualitative approaches to the exploration of human experience, developing methods of relating man's experience in the world with their perceptions and views of the progression of their existence. Like Freud, May recognized that there is a connection between the conflict individuals feel in their experiences and their responses, including what May viewed as their courage and capacity for future development.

May related psychological functioning to elements that frequently come into play when assessing the meaning of existence: the assessment of personal freedom, the ability to make decisions, the capacity for alienation, and living life authentically (Grogan 143). May recognized that the progression of motivational factors toward the achievement of an essential sense of self was frequently the cause of anxiety and this anxiety occurred in the presence of disparities between capacity and action or between action and authenticity. Subsequently, May supported the belief that the progression of man's identify was shaped by the angst created in attempting to meet foundational needs.

✖ Maslow

Though American psychologist Abraham Maslow (1908–1970) is often described as a humanistic psychologist, his view of the process by which individuals seek self-actualization and his reference of existential principles places him in the scope of discourse on existential psychoanalytical processes. Maslow created his holistic-dynamic theory to explain how individuals work through forces that impact self-determination and how motivations drive actions. Maslow believed that conflict and choice arise over specific types of motivational factors and individuals cannot move toward a greater assessment of tangential needs if essential or base needs go unmet.

Motivation for self-actualization or the ability to answer the questions of meaning and existence come second to addressing lower-level needs, including hunger, safety, love, and esteem.

Erskine, Moursund and Trautmann described eight relational needs that are foundationally linked to Abraham Maslow's hierarchy: security, valuing, acceptance, mutuality, self-definition, initiation by the other person, and the need to express love. Maslow adapted a holistic and existential perspective on the progression of the psyche by defining a connection between self-actualization and psychoanalytical processes. Like Rollo May, Maslow believed that psychotherapeutic process had to be dynamic and directly in alignment with the progression of essential needs. Maslow criticized Freud's perspective about the foundations of behaviors and instead asserted that there is a hierarchy of needs that defines how an individual acts upon drives. Individuals place an emphasis on their essential needs first, then their motivations toward greater self-actualization, and then finally an evaluation of how they can support the self-actualization of others. Like May, Maslow applied evaluations of case studies and assessments of individual psychological process to the progressing of his ideal of self-actualization. From an existential perspective, self-actualization for Maslow was the ultimate realization of human experience (Berger 29).

❧ Erikson

Erik Erikson (1902–1994) was born in Germany but developed his views of psychological functioning in response to Freud's views in the early part of the twentieth century and as an extension of research and professional development in the Ivy League schools of the United States. Though Erikson's stages of psychological and psychosocial development related a structural paradigm to psychoanalysis, his theories were beneficial in understanding the progression of development over the life span. It was Erikson's contention, for example, that psychosocial development reflected on elements like trust, personal control, and the development of happiness. Like Freud, Erikson linked early relationship formation, especially the relationship between mother and child, to the creation of trust that has an underlying impact through the life span. Erikson's earliest stage of development reflects the trust or mistrust that develops between care provider (usually mother) and child, including the child's belief that the mother may leave but will return. Trust formation at the early stage of development in childhood can impact relationships later in life and determine the successful integration of trust as a means of assessing psychological balance.

Erikson related the process of pursuing personal control to the second stage of development, when children assert control over self-care skills, including eating, toileting, talking, and moving. During this stage, independence is frequently asserted with an overly aggressive sense of capabilities and caregiver or parental roles are often defined by protecting children from their own efforts at personal control. Learning the essential skill of being both independent and dependent at the same time becomes an important lesson that children take with them later in life.

Though Erikson's sixth stage of development reflects the goal of adults in pursing romantic love and relationships, this is not the stage that is always reflective of periods of happiness or the ability to achieve happiness. In fact, this stage is often marked by emotional angst and conflicts and efforts to repeatedly manage conflicts. In young adulthood, the formation of relationships and family often occur that can be both the source of happiness and the source of conflict (Erikson's Stages of Development 1). Stage seven of Erikson's eight developmental stages is actually the stage most likely to promote contentment and happiness as a function of adult activities (Erikson's Stages of Development 1). Adults between the ages of forty and sixty-five are frequently involved with supporting family and promoting the gains of others, an element that frequently fosters a sense of well-being and happiness that corresponds with contributing to society as a whole.

Like Maslow, Erikson believed that the progression from one stage to the next required a level of completion or the successful integration of principles, and this included an understanding of the movement of self through the life span. Though not specifically attuned to the concept of self-actualization, Erikson posed the stage approach to recognizing the movement toward the achievement of each step in the progression of the authentic human experiences.

❊ Jung and Allport

Many theorists, including Swiss psychologist Carl Jung (1875–1961) and American psychologist George Allport (1897–1967), recognized that psychological development may include a view of a measurable set of traits, some of which may be present from a very early age but also include experiential influences that shift over time. Personality describes a measurable set of traits within a given time period, but those traits and the expression of those traits can be impacted by psychosocial functioning and interpersonal interactions. Personal development can be influenced by environmental factors including the impacts of home life on early childhood development, both of which define a contextualized connection between psychological functioning and real experiences. These views are in alignment with the connection between the research of these two humanistic psychologists and the creation of a humanistic-existential approach that contextualizes human development.

Jung's conceptual view of self and the link between development of the human psyche and experiential elements was in alignment with the humanist-existential approach. At the same time, Jung also placed the context of human development within an interrelational construct, maintaining the importance of social connections. Jung's subsequent assertions about the importance of the psyche and the presence of a collective unconscious determined a separation from some of the more traditional existentialist perspectives. At the same time, Jung's perspective, including his assertion about the nature of archetypes and the presence of a collective unconscious, created their own set of essential questions about the nature and meaning of man's existence.

Allport supported the importance of self-actualization

as a component of his existential perspective. Allport maintained that factors like intelligence could have a substantial impact on the expression of sense of self and could play a role in how a person perceives their capacity for self-actualization. Allport argued that intelligence can influence expressions of personality and capability, just as temperament can determine how capability plays out in interactions with others. Allport maintained that struggles commonly emerge when attempting to create a cohesive view of the progression of traits that influence capabilities. As individuals move through the life span, the culmination of elements can influence how individuals assess their self-worth (Allport 284). Allport argued, though, also identified the importance of accepting the finite nature of the human mind and the human psyche. Correspondingly, personality and humanistic psychology promoted a sense of understanding of the characteristics of a psyche and the personal forms, individualized as a progression of self that emerged.

❋ Carl Rogers

Though American psychologist Carl Rogers (1902–1987) is often viewed as a humanistic psychologist, his approach to identifying self and relating the concept of self to the progression of human identify is based on humanistic, existential, and phenomenological components that are valuable in creating a psychoanalytic praxis. Rogers developed his approach based on the belief that there did not need to be a divide between humanistic psychology and existential process. Rogers applied rigorous standards of research to the development of his existential perspective, including his theories regarding the nature of self and the impacts of the therapeutic environment on individual process (Vincent 3).

Rogers developed a person-centered therapeutic approach based on humanistic and existential principles in response to the long-standing psychoanalytical approach that was fostered by theorists like Freud. Rogers rejected the belief that therapists should lead or direct the approach or that they should be placed in the position of problem-solver and identified methods through which therapists could support the work done by the client. This directly challenged a body of work that had been in place by Freudian and Neo-Freudian psychologists and reflected the importance of the therapeutic relationship within the exploration of the psyche (Capuzzi and Gross 6).

Rogers defined a method for achieving an atmosphere that was conducive to healing by a "nondirective method" that totally avoided questions, interpretation, suggestions, advice, or other directive techniques. Rather, it relied exclusively on a process of carefully listening to the client, accepting the client for who he or she is—no matter how confused or antisocial that might be at the moment—and skillfully reflecting back the client's feelings. (Kirschenbaum 116)

Rogers's person-centered approach extended from his belief in individual process and the role of the therapist as a facilitator in supporting self-actualization. Rogers's theories on the individual and the therapeutic process linked both to existential and phenomenological principles led to his views of nineteen essential propositions. These propositions set the foundation for Rogers's views and related his belief in the role of the therapist in providing support in relation to a person-centered approach. These propositions included the belief that individuals are constantly changing and responding to their world of which they are the center, and individual reality is based on how an individual reacts to the world. At the same time, Rogers believed that individuals are constantly striving toward self-actualization and that individuals have a constant drive to enhance their experiences within their own environment. The progression of self, including the development of personality characteristics, is related to both to the internal frame of reference of the individual and the experience that influence individual development.

Like other humanistic psychologists, Rogers also viewed the importance of self-actualization in realizing goals and in creating goal directed behaviors. Values and experiences are linked to the focus on self and the belief that the individual will move toward the greater attainment of personal goals. As an individual has different experiences, these experiences are interpreted and integrated into the sense of self, ignored if they do not apply or have significance that can be perceived, or denied or distorted if they do not have perceived benefit.

From a psychological standpoint, the individual interpretation of experiences becomes an essential part of understanding individual perceptions. Psychological dysfunction occurs when individuals are unable to understand the significance of experiences or when they ignore the impacts of external stressors on psychological function. Experiences that are in conflict with an individual's self-perception or self-actualization may be perceived as a threat to the individuals, and a level of rigid response can occur that leads to denial of the impacts.

Individual perceptions then are structured around value systems, experiences, and the distorted symbolism that is placed on the interpretation of information.

As a component of the response to individual needs, Rogers defined his person-centered approach around understanding the foundations of individual's perceptions and experiences and the responses to phenomenological conditions without placing specific value judgments on the experiences of the individual. Rogers identified the need for unconditional positive regard as an essential component of the therapeutic relationship, defining the role of the therapist as an individual supporting the goal of self-actualization (Corey 170).

Rogers maintained that within the scope of this concept, therapists needed to understand that all people are innately good and have the potential for realizing this. Rogers supported the belief that people are "kind, concerned, friendly and effective" if experience and support focus on self-actualization (Holme 646). Contrary to other therapeutic approaches, Rogers did not believe that therapy was inherently created to solve problems or relieve dysfunction but to support a client's capacity for coping with current issues and addressing potential problems that can arise in the future.

The concept of actualization is a component of the

existential elements supported in Rogers's view, and this was as the main goal of the therapeutic interaction. Rogers believed that each child is born with an innate ability or drive called an "actualizing tendency" that, given the correct foundation, could result in the development of the ideal self.

Rogers supported the belief that people who were actualized have a similar set of characteristics, including the following:

- an openness to experience
- a trust in themselves
- an internal source of evaluation
- a willingness to continue growing (Corey 170)

It was Rogers's contention that the process of self-actualization is often subverted in individual experiences and that during the course of experiences, individuals move away from this natural process. As a result, psychological issues extend from what Rogers recognized as the development of incongruence between a person's potential and their experience. Person-centered therapy then is applied to the methods to reduce the conflict a person experiences that move them away from self-actualization.

The concept of actualization is based on the belief that when a client seeks interaction in the therapeutic environment, he or she does so because of a "feeling of basic helplessness, powerlessness, and an inability to make decisions or effectively direct their own lives." When this individual can assess the role that they play in these emotions and identify their actions related to this role, they are better able to develop self-understanding and apply this in the therapeutic process. The interaction between the therapist and client is based on the progression of interactions that support self-awareness and self-healing, by empowering the individual to take responsibility for the process of change. The communications and interactions between the therapist and the client provide a basis for developing trust and promoting self-healing through the application of unconditional positive regard. This concept is based on the therapist's ability to take an empathetic approach to interactions with the client and to apply this empathy to the verbal messages and nonverbal cues that are used in the therapy session.

Rogers (1995) argued that a full understanding empathy was necessary in creating a specific therapeutic response. The following extension of a definition of empathy was created by Rogers to address previous limitations. Empathy is the process by which a person is entering the private, perceptual world of the other … being sensitive, moment by moment, to the changing felt meanings which flow in this other person … sensing meanings of which he or she is scarcely aware … communicating your sensings of the person's world.

Rogers recognized that it is not enough for a therapist utilizing this approach to tell a person that he or she is worthy, good, and whole; the therapist has to help the person in the process of self-actualization to either realize that these elements are present or to support the individual in developing them (Holme 646). Unconditional positive regard is the basis for the interactions that leads a patient to "reevaluate, accept, and finally integrate his own feelings within the self" as the client struggles to make his attitudes about himself more congruent with experience. Rogers recognized that therapists can take on two different roles that can hinder this process; they can either be distant and unhelpful or they can guide/direct a person through a process that may lack authenticity. Rogers believed that therapists and clients should be in psychological contact with each other and that by doing this, a support mechanism can be in place that helps one move toward greater self-actualization. Subsequently, Rogers believed that the empathic contact that therapists must foster is linked to the capacity of the therapist to support a person-centered approach and to integrate practical aspects of this therapeutic ideal in the creation of a professional relationship.

Rogers introduced some very specific views of the development of the psyche, the identification of self-concept, and the progression of psychopathology. Foremost, Rogers assessed human development in relation to specific principles and interconnected components rather than taking a stage approach that is common in developmental or cognitive psychology. Individuals move through a process of self-development in which interactions with others plays a role in shaping perceptions of self. It was Rogers's contention that the development of personality was an ongoing process that may take many shifts over the life span.

Subsequently, Rogers commonly utilized a range of terms relating to the identification of self and the progression of personality, including self-experience, self-concept, and self-structure. Rogers maintained that these concepts all revolved around a "conceptual gestalt" that referred to the characteristics of "I" or "me" as well as the way in which these characteristics were brought together and the "values attached to these perceptions." Correspondingly, the progression of awareness of the gestalt and the constant changes that it is subjected to relate to the process of personality formation. "The term self or self-concept is more likely to be used when we are talking of the person's view of himself, self-structure when we are looking at this gestalt from an external frame of reference." Rogers recognized that within the scope of self-concept, there could also be an ideal of a self-concept that an individual hoped to obtain, and that this would be described as the actualization of the "ideal self."

Rogers believed that there is a foundational connection between regard, both positive and negative, and the capacity of an individual to become their ideal self. The "regard complex" described by Rogers was initially constructed by Standal "as all those self-experiences, together with their interrelationships, which the individual discriminates as being related to positive regards of a particular social other." Subsequently, there is a potent connection between the positive regard demonstrated to a child and the development of particular strengths and levels of resiliency. If a parent shows positive regard for their child, the child will strengthen behaviors or characteristics that are most likely to result in positive regard. If a child experiences negative regard, they are less likely to be able to demonstrate characteristics that are linked to positive regard.

Optimal development or the achieving of the ideal self is linked to methods for achieving congruence, first between self and experience. Rogers maintained that the state of congruence between self and experience is identified when "self-experiences are accurately symbolized, and are included in the self-concept in this accurately symbolized form." If a person demonstrated congruence in all forms of self-experience, the person would be what Rogers deemed a

> fully functioning person … If it is true of some specific aspect of experience, such as the individual's experience in a given relationship or in a given moment in time, then we can say that the individual is to this degree in a state of congruence …

In achieving a fully functioning state though, Rogers also maintained that individuals must demonstrate a level of openness to experiences.

A fully functioning person also demonstrates psychological adjustment or the assimilation of self at a symbolic level "into the gestalt of the self-structure."

In addition, extensionality is a component of the fully functioning person and reflects the focus on congruence as an essential part of this process. Individuals must trust in their understanding of the nature of abstraction and the impact it has on individual perception. Finally, Rogers asserted the importance of maturity in relating to the progression of congruence toward a full functioning individual. A person has reached a state of maturity if the person

> perceives realistically and in an extensional manner, is not defensive, accepts the responsibility of being different from others, accepts responsibility for his own behavior, evaluates experiences … changes his evaluations … on the basis of new evidence … accepts others … prizes himself and prizes others.

In addressing the development of true self through the progression of congruence, Rogers also had to address the idea of incongruence and its impacts, especially in relation to psychopathology. Individuals are vulnerable and may be unable to be self-actualizing in the presence of incongruence. Individuals may not always be aware of the state of incongruence, but Rogers identified it in relation to the following elements:

> potential vulnerability to anxiety, threat, and disorganization. If a significant new experience demonstrates the discrepancy so clearly that it must be consciously perceived, then the individual will be threatened, and his concept of self-disorganized by this contradictory and inassimilable experience.

More concisely, Rogers recognized the presence of incongruence when discrepancies existed between the actual self and the ideal self and between the individual that the person has become and the person they should or wish to be.

Incongruence can lead to defensiveness and to denial or distortion as a result of the inability to self-actualize. This can result in the presence of anxiety and threats to congruence and the development of situations in which dishonesty and defensiveness become a prevalent part of interactions. Anxiety, in Rogers's view, was based on the development of "a state of uneasiness or tension" with an unknown cause, which is generally the result of the presence of an external frame of reference and from the presence of incongruence. "Anxiety is the response of the organism to the 'subception' that such discrepancy may enter awareness, thus forcing a change in self-concept." Rogers maintained that maladjustment or psychopathology emerged as a result of a lack of awareness in individual rationality and when defenses or distorted self-concept influence decision-making. Essentially, a person develops dysfunctional traits when their decisions "are inconsistent with the dictates of their organismic evaluations. The organismic valuing process in individuals enables them to make value judgments and choices based on their sensory and visceral experiences and organismic processing of situations" (Thomas 200). Individuals can avoid dysfunction by trusting their organismic value process and aiming toward becoming a fully functioning being in the world.

⚘ Aging and Existentialism

Existential principles maintained by many of the theorists presented can be related in regard to the progression of aging. Two elements that come into play significantly include the importance placed on the context or experiences through which the psyche progresses and the application of meaning to determining methods for coping. Existing research supports the argument that as people age, they seek social support and apply strategies toward self-actualization as a means of coping with their psychological and physiological changes.

Individuals use a variety of strategies or coping mechanisms to manage stress that can have positive and negative ramifications. Many of these are developed as a result of social learning and the coping behaviors learned within our individual social cultures (Laureate Education 2). For example, if a person is a part of a religious community that utilizes faith-based messages in response to stress resulting from medical emergencies or illness, this strategy might influence the choices of a person as they age. Correspondingly, individuals with significant social support mechanisms in place often define their process of self-actualization in relation to these elements.

Delongis and Holtzman maintained that social support mechanisms play a significant role in the response to stress social networks and support provide a foundation for integrating coping mechanisms in the presence of significant life changes and this is an underlying defense for the use of group support programming for individuals who develop significant health problems (166). Individuals who have support systems in place, including prosocial family systems and/or supportive social relationships, often demonstrate more effective coping approaches (Delongis and Holtzman 166). Research also indicates though that the same social factors that determine the effectiveness of social support mechanisms in coping with stress can also support the use of problematic behaviors, including denial of the progression of aging or lack of meaningfulness to life at the end of life (Berg et al., 239).

Coping with Aging

Problem-focused, emotion-focused, and biology-focused are three different types of coping mechanisms that can be used to address a range of stressors and are often considered when determining approaches to therapeutic interventions. An effective problem-focused approach would be to identify the source of stress and remove it. For example, if a person is experiencing stress over a parent's interactions and comments about a health issue, the individual could refrain from contact with the parent until the health issue is resolved. For people who are aging though, this kind of approach cannot be applied to a problem that is not going to change.

An emotion-focused approach is the process of readjusting perspective in order to reduce stress and change the emotional response to an issue and is in alignment in many ways with the existential and humanistic approaches supported by Rogers. For example, when a person has a serious illness, it may be impossible to change the diagnosis, but the person could choose self-actualization or empowerment rather than feeling defeated or stressed by the diagnosis. This could include focusing on positive elements, including fostering a close relationship with friends and family.

A biology-focused coping mechanism is the use of techniques or strategies that have a physiological impact to address stress. For example, mediation, deep-breathing techniques, and even physical exercise are all approaches that can be used to reduce stress. The key to the effectiveness of these strategies is that there has to be a connection between the approach and reductions in the stress response and a positive impact of the behavior.

Ineffective approaches can occur using each of these techniques. For example, an ineffective problem-focused approach would be to attempt to manage the stress around a spouse's end-stage illness by focusing on the problem. Because the problem is not going to change (the spouse's health is not going to improve), attempts to change the problem will not have a positive impact (Laureate Education 2). Subsequently, the application of an approach to address this issue requires an identification of strategies to address declining health, meaning, and self-actualization while also creating effective goals for continued participation in the process of living.

Rogers's mode of therapeutic action related an understanding of two primary concepts that were distinctly connected: congruence and therapeutic presence. Though other components of the therapeutic relationship, including empathic response, shaped the essential components of person-centered therapy, Rogers believed that each therapist could develop an exact method for applying empathic response in developing cohesiveness within the counseling process. The components of the therapeutic process that were essential to progress were congruence and therapeutic presence, and these influenced the actions of both the client and therapist.

Rogers believed that this essential component of the therapeutic relationship was what defined the attitudes and feelings that directed the process. Specifically, Rogers and colleagues (1967) maintained that the therapist must demonstrate the openness of "being the feelings and attitudes which at the moment are flowing with him." The existential process and role of the therapist are to support the client in developing a sense of "inherent worth" and in defining personal interactions based on shared value (Kirschenbaum 6). The unification that occurs in the therapeutic process between the client and therapist is essential in facilitating therapeutic change. Central to this process is the capacity of the therapist to demonstrate appropriate responses and regard for the client. Knox and Cooper maintained that the ability of the therapist to demonstrate presence in the relationship is vital to the capacity to facilitate for the client and to provide a safe environment "in which the client can confront her problems and act upon her discoveries." The focus on a therapist's ability to be present, to feel immersed in the relationship, and to have the capacity to ground the client are all factors that have been related in a number of research studies of the response of therapists to the ideals of an existential approach.

❊ Impact of Fear

When considering the impacts of research into the application of a praxis for therapeutic response to the needs of an aging population, the conceptual view of fear, especially death fear, comes into play in relation to meaning, existence, and the development of the psyche. Death fear is a relatively general term that is often used interchangeably with the concept of death anxiety, with some distinct differences (Feifel and Branscomb 282). The term "death fear" reflects a contemplative process by which the individuals assess and reassess their perspectives on dying and death. Some elements of death fear include fear of the unknown, fear of pain, having "unfinished business," and fear of nonexistence (Feifel and Branscomb 283). This type of contemplating and rationale process reflects the view that individuals facing death experience a significant level of angst related to the end of life in a very rationale and experiential manner (Feifel and Nagy 278).

In contrast, individuals facing the end of life may also experience death anxiety, which is a much less tangible process by which individuals demonstrate both psychological and physiological manifestations of anxiety that are in direct alignment with angst related to the end of life. In relation to existential theorists and views on psychopathology, Freud's belief that individuals process a significant amount of angst-related experiences subconsciously fits with the definition of death anxiety. While many people may express acceptance of or awareness of paradigmatic views on death, the afterlife, and even spiritual believes, fear of death is universal, even when it is not consciously verbalized. Death anxiety occurs when a person cannot match their beliefs or views on death with the actual process of dying.

The existential view on death fear relates to the views of Frankl, May, and Rogers regarding the importance of self-actualization. Death fear and death anxiety that last for prolonged periods of time often stem from a fear of the lack of self-actualization or the belief that a person has not achieved a level of meaning in his or her life. Erikson maintained the importance of identifying the progression of the psyche in stages that allow for an assessment of the nature of achievement over the life span. For many, self-actualization extends from the belief that the individual has progressed through the stages of development, the end product of which was a life that appeared of value to self and/or others.

Though life interrupted early by death is often seen as a negative element because the individual was unable to progress through the life cycle, aging is the process by which individuals navigate the life process, the end product of which is death. Though this is a very blunt perspective on the reality of life, many of the existential theorists, from Heidegger and Sartre to Rogers, believed that it was important to acknowledge the very concrete nature of death as a part of the progression of life. Self-actualization then extends from the belief that life was worth living and that at the end meaning could be derived from that life. The concept of self-actualization extends from a Socratic principle that the "unexamined life is not worth living" (Socrates, *Apology* 38). Feifel and Nagel maintained that this kind of perspective is essential to understanding why some individuals develop death fear and death anxiety while others do not. One very clear explanation may extend from the Rogerian view of self-actualization and the belief that death acceptance comes upon the completion of life rather than the cessation of life.

Klug and Boss maintained that there were two central components to any process that supports death acceptance or the positive view of death as completion, rather than the termination, of a life process. These two elements are the ability to confront (identify and rationally view) death and to integrate an understanding of the meaning of death in relation to emotional, psychological, and psychosocial functioning (Klug and Boss 907).

✖ Conflicting Views on Death

One of the central problems in creating a response to death fear and death anxiety linked to an existential psychoanalytical praxis is that there is a conflicted cultural view on death and a lack of cohesiveness in views of death process. When people take the life of a pet suffering from a terminal disease or in incredible pain, the action is deemed humane and prolonging the animal's life might be perceived as a selfish act on the part of the animal owner. Though we afford this kind of kindness and humane treatment to our pets, we do not give the same option to their human counterparts. If a person has a terminal disease or is living with incredible pain, human life is valued above the humane treatment of the individual. As a result, death is more than just the completion of a life cycle; it is frequently viewed an event to be set aside, sequestered, and removed from valid discourse.

In the past, death was a process that was fairly simple; individuals simply stopped breathing for whatever reason and cell necrosis quickly ensued. Bodily functions stopped and brain activity ceased, all of which define end of life. The advent of technologies that can prolong life in the presence of a lack of independent bodily functions and even brain activity creates a whole new set of parameters for assessing death and dying (Feifel and Boss 907). Dying can be a prolonged, painful, and often disjointed process in which technological advances determine the continuation of life rather than actually living it. Death used to be a process requiring family participation and end-of-life care that is no longer so simply defied. Contemporary medical practices apply a variety of standards to assessing both care at the end of life and the determination of death (Beach and Morrison 2057).

Part of this extends from the desire to prolong life and part of this extends from the desire to take the mess out of death. Increasingly, families are participating in acts that reflect the sequestration of death and methods to take the pain, discomfort, and tragedy out of the event (McKenzie 119). The process of dying no longer occurs simply in the home but also in long-term care facilities and hospitals, and even the aging and dying have access to medical technologies to prolong life (Stanley and Wise 947). The message provided to people in the process of aging is that death is an event inherently to be prevented, and modern medicine, with its many complicated elements, can help to hold off death as long as possible. As people age and live longer and longer, the progression of the life cycle extends, as does the period of time during which older adults assess and reassess their purpose and meaningfulness. The cultural views of death and the progression of technologies in the modern world have led to the need for an existential psychoanalytic praxis to address the needs of elderly experiencing a range of fear responses to the potentiality of death.

❉ Summary

There was a broad range of theoretical foundational studies for the application of an existential praxis for addressing end-of-life experiences in the elderly. The background of existential perspectives provided a substantive body of support for the connection between assessments of self-actualization and methods for addressing fear and death anxiety. Carl Rogers provided an example of the application of the existential exploration of self-actualization that was utilized in the creation of a foundational psychoanalytic praxis for use with the elderly. This corresponded with the connection between variables that influenced end-of-life perspectives, including different views on life, meaningfulness, and death. The progression of this literature review reflected the importance of creating a backdrop from which the praxis was developed.

CHAPTER 3
RESEARCH METHODS

THE RESEARCH METHOD FOR ASSESSING A psychoanalytic existential praxis for support for elderly populations was based on the use of a mixed method approach. The research questions identified in the introduction of the study related both qualitative and quantitative data collection opportunities with the goals of creating a body of research that addresses both client and practitioner views of the praxis and the potential methods for addressing end-of-life conflicts. The following questions were used to guide the qualitative assessments of the feasibility and implementation of an existential psychoanalytic praxis for use with elderly patients:

- How feasible is the application of the proposed existential psychoanalytic praxis to the process of care for elderly patients?

- How successful were the therapists at implementing the existential psychoanalytic praxis, and how successful was the praxis in improving self-awareness and reducing anxiety?

In order to gain insight into the implications of the research question for elderly patients/clients seeking treatment in a therapeutic environment, the following quantitative research question was developed: After implementing the newly designed existential psychoanalytic praxis for a period of five weeks, how effective is the approach in meeting the needs of elderly clients/patients? Specifically, will these individuals demonstrate improvements in regard to their specific individual goals, reductions in anxiety responses, and reductions in death fear?

❋ Research Philosophy

The research philosophy for this study was based on an interpretivist view that applied a systematic evaluation of content derived from a focus group, interviews, and a questionnaire survey utilizing a thematic grouping approach (Savin-Baden and Major 135). This philosophy supports the belief that in therapeutic interactions, therapists can apply an existential psychoanalytic praxis that promotes a reflective and culturally maintained perspective that can be interpreted, understood, and experienced by elderly clients. This provides a foundation for interpreting variations in the therapeutic process and the implications for supporting this type of approach in the clinical setting.

The philosophical underpinnings were supported in existential and phenomenological approaches applying interpretivism as a foundation for analysis of data (Remler and Van Ryzin 440). This philosophical view related the importance of studying individuals and collecting data in a natural setting and providing a contextual view of narrative data collected through a qualitative approach. Because the research focus of this study related significantly to the role that individual self-actualization plays in defining the therapeutic process, motivation, and response to change, this approach aligns the research focus and philosophical underpinning.

❋ Purpose and Process

The purpose of this study was to evaluate the views of therapists and aging clients in an outpatient mental health clinic to determine the benefits of an existential psychoanalytical praxis in addressing specific issues for aging populations. This study applied a mixed method approach to the assessment of specific perceptions regarding the use of the praxis and to determine whether the approach supports beneficial change for aging clients. This research proposal was based on a nonexperimental design that integrated views presented in the current literature with assessments made through the use of interviews, a focus group response scenario, and questionnaire surveys of both therapists and clients in an outpatient setting.

❋ Setting

The setting for this study was an outpatient clinic in an urban setting that provides outpatient support services for a large population of elderly adults (over the age of sixty-five). The organization was selected based on the willingness of the administration to self-assess for need and identifying the need for a new praxis to improve outcomes for elderly patients with end-of-life care needs. In addition, the agency was selected based on their willingness to participate in the assessments of both clients and therapists. The use of an organization in a large urban setting was selected in order to ensure that a diverse population could be located and that the participants might have a varied perspective that could inform assessments of death fear, death anxiety, and end-of-life care scenarios.

❇ Sample Selection

The primary sample population in this study consisted of subjects selected from the clients and practitioners (therapists) in the selected setting, with a total subject population of twenty patient subjects and ten therapists. This study looked at the outcomes of a questionnaire survey of demographic features and a survey of questions on death fear, death anxiety, and self-actualization perspectives. This study included a request for participation from the organization, request for permission to conduct the study from the administration, and a waiver for participants, all of which must be received prior to the initiation of the study. (See appendices.) Further, administrative staff was also required to demonstrate a willingness to participate, and assessment of willingness, including a needs assessment, was conducted prior to the selection of the agency.

The sampling was designed to coordinate the protocols for the study with the necessary subject population requirements. In order to select certain available subjects and conduct both surveys and a focus group to respond to questions, convenience sampling was necessary. In addition, it should also be recognized that the process of evaluating the subjects, in the clinical setting and providing for responses was an element of consideration in evaluating the willingness for participation, and administrator responses were taken into consideration as a part of the selection process for the testing environment as a whole.

In order to effectively delineate the subjects based on possible gender, cultural, or age biases, demographic considerations for this study include the following:

- age
- gender
- educational attainment
- ethnicity/race
- socioeconomic status

The research identified measures to protect the rights of human subjects via the application of informed consent and the review of the consent process. Because human subjects were utilized and data was collected from these subjects, informed consent was just one component of the protocols for the use in this research study. (See appendices.) The researcher followed the protocols set by the university in regard to the use of human subjects, the approval process, and reviews of the ethics of human research.

The study did not pose any significant risks to the participant population being studied and provided a body of data that support improvements to the process of care for the client population. The study outcomes were provided to the study participants and organization at the conclusion of the study in order to support mechanisms for change.

❊ Materials/Instruments

The primary instrument for this study is a questionnaire survey provided to clients and therapists about their understanding of and feelings about death, death anxiety, death fear, and the existential psychoanalytical praxis. This instrument was created to provide comparative data that was evaluated relative to the thematic focal point of the study: the identification of the best approach for addressing client needs related to counseling surrounding end-of-life experiences.

A chart was utilized that includes the numeric data collected for the questions in the survey. The data from this instrument was provided in a narrative format. This helped to identify any significant functional or thematic findings that impacted perceptions of the major themes and the impacts of the approach. Narrative data was compiled from a focus group specifically to address the major themes presented in some of the open-ended questions in the survey, including the following:

- How successful were the therapists at implementing the existential psychoanalytic praxis?
- How successful was the praxis in improving self-awareness and reducing anxiety?
- Has the questionnaire missed any important elements related to counseling, death anxiety, or death fear? If so, what are they?

These open-ended questions—one that looks at the specific limitations that a person might perceive in the counseling process and the other that reflects potential limitations to the survey instrument—were designed to help to inform the outcomes of the study and ensure that a clear depiction of the therapeutic approach was related.

❧ Data Collection Process

Each participant was provided with a disclosure statement and was required to sign informed consent prior to participation. The coded demographic questionnaire was provided and responses were noted before distributing the broader questionnaire or participation in the focus group for client participants. Subjects will be asked to take the questionnaires independently and to turn them in anonymously, utilizing a coded envelope to ensure anonymity.

Data collected from the research subjects as evaluated and provided in a narrative format and the information was assessed to see if any major messages or themes appeared in relation to gender bias. Major themes were identified and the information was provided in a narrative format within these themes from the questionnaire responses.

The results for this study were based on the following criteria for data collection: The data was collected by the survey utilizing varied questions. By promoting varied responses through the instrument, it was the hope of the researcher to bring about the greatest level of response from the subjects. The researcher instructed participants to provide as little discussion around the survey as possible. They were also instructed to take the surveys in private settings to allow for the greatest confidentiality in response.

The researcher collected all the data until a sufficient number of responses was received and it was determined that no other responses would be forthcoming, and two different sessions were allocated for assessments of response status in a clinical setting. The researcher then discussed the findings with a statistician and created a document representing the data in a quantitative format.

The data was processed through the use of SPSS software, and the statistical data was provided in graphs and charts based on the outcomes of the data sets produced.

A focus group was conducted, and participants were asked to respond to a set of focus group questions. The information collected from this group was recorded and transcribed and information was provided in narrative format. The focus group was an interview process that took place collectively and assessed the views of ten elderly clients. These individuals were brought together in a group and asked open-ended questions about the nature of their experiences with the psychoanalytic praxis based on existentialism. They were specifically asked to relate their views on the progression of change in relation to their views of death anxiety and death fear. The role of the researcher in the focus group was to ask open-ended questions and facilitate the group in discussing the specific questions that were introduced. As in the semistructured interviews, the focus group information was recorded and field notes were taken to ensure the accuracy of information collected through this process.

Interview data was also collected from the therapist participants through open-ended questions, and responses were assessed for any significant recurring thematic properties.

❦ Data Analysis

Client and therapist participants were given ample opportunity to respond to survey questionnaires and submit their responses. The data analysis process occurred in two parts: the assessment of inputted statistical data through a software program like SPSS, as described above, and the subsequent evaluation of the data with outcomes produced in narrative form from the current literature, interviews, and focus group narratives (Remler and Van Ryzin 440). Because of the nonexperimental nature of this research study, the data collected from the survey was used in conjunction with the secondary data collected in narrative format to determine the impacts of a specific approach to exploring issues related to end-of-life care.

❋ Potential Limits of the Methodology

Survey designs are often used to assess the views of a large subject population. These survey approaches can include cross-sectional surveys of a selected population or longitudinal studies in which a questionnaire can be utilized or data can be collected through structured interviews and information from the sample can be generalized (Creswell 14). In each of these types of studies, the data collected is finite and represents the specific parameters of time and study constructs. As a result, quantitative research is commonly viewed as a single snapshot of data that is collected at a specific time and is only applicable in relation to the understanding of its finite nature. The size of the population utilized for this study was better suited for a qualitative research study, so this type of study has limits in relation to both the potential presence for researcher bias and limitations in generalizability in relation to the quantitative elements of the study (Creswell 14). The mixed methodology was used to address this issue (Remler and Van Ryzin 128).

Specifically, the information collected through interviews and a focus group in the clinical setting was beneficial in influencing how the research outcomes were perceived. The quantitative data provided was limited in relation to statistical significance because of the relatively small subject populations and the inability to reach data saturation. The combined approach to creating a thematic view of the data was based on the belief that it would help to ensure that an adequate body of data was collected and analyzed for the purpose of addressing the research questions.

❋ Data Analysis and Presentation

The thematic grouping approach that was utilized was based on four fundamental steps: the identification of themes that repeat in the data; collection of similar content grouped to form concepts; the identification of grouped concepts to demonstrate categories; and the utilization of categories in the formation of a theoretical perspective applied, analyzed, or compared with other research. The data was collected separately for interviews and collectively for the focus group, and the coding occurred based on the sum total of the narrative data collected.

The data was presented in table format that identifies major themes. Individual comments or statements that promote specific thematic areas are included in the presentation of the data. This means that the data appeared in both narrative and table formats to add to the ease of discussing the findings in relation to the current literature.

❦ Summary

The methods presented provide a basis for understanding the factors influencing perceptions of death fear, death anxiety, and the use of an existential psychoanalytic praxis for elderly clients. This study underscores the importance of this process for determining interactions in the clinical setting and for potential improvements in the approaches for addressing death anxiety and death fear as people progress through the life span.

CHAPTER 4
RESULTS AND DISCUSSION

THE RESEARCH FINDINGS WERE GROUPED BY demographic findings, thematic findings related to each of the research questions, and views on the use of the proposed existential psychoanalytic praxis. As a part of the evaluative and interpretive nature of the research process, each of these segments of information was assessed in relation to findings regarding the impacts of this type of approach related in the literature. The findings were presented in the form of tables and charts as well as discussion on the major themes and group information presented in narrative format.

❀ Study Demographics

The student demographic data was provided as a foundation for addressing any potential factors that could influence the study outcomes and was provided for informational purposes. The demographic data collected for the study includes the study participant data, including information collected from the personal questionnaire provided in the appendix. The narrative elements of the demographic data include reflections of some of the therapists in relation to their client populations and the best approaches for treatment as perceived by the therapist. For example, one therapist identified specific trends in recent years, including a growing focus on longevity and the importance of medical technology in care for the elderly. This information was provided as a supplement to the narrative data to show the potential factors influencing views on life, death, and death fear and death anxiety.

The data presented in figure 1 reflects the ethnic/racial composition of the subject population. This date demonstrates the benefits of utilizing a study facility in an urban population because of the representative diversity of the subject population.

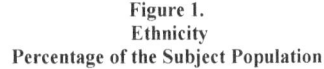

Figure 1.
Ethnicity
Percentage of the Subject Population

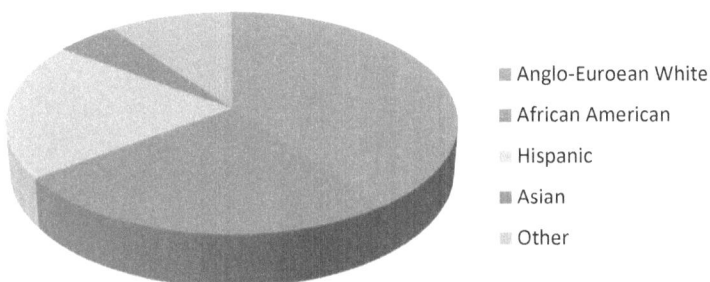

- Anglo-Euroean White
- African American
- Hispanic
- Asian
- Other

This indicates a slight difference from the narrative data provided by one of the therapists about the composition of the client population, though this may be in part because of the interactions with the therapist and specific segments of the population. One therapist maintained that their facility worked with a much higher percentage of African Americans than in the general population, though this did not seem to be indicated in the subject population selected for participation in the study.

The data collected in figure 2 represents the level of educational attainment for the study populations, including both clients and therapists. This information was collected to ensure that the questionnaires utilized and the focus group information matched the expected literacy levels of the subject participants and also provided information about potential impacts of information presented in the study if subjects did not meet minimum educational requirements that could impact their ability for full participation.

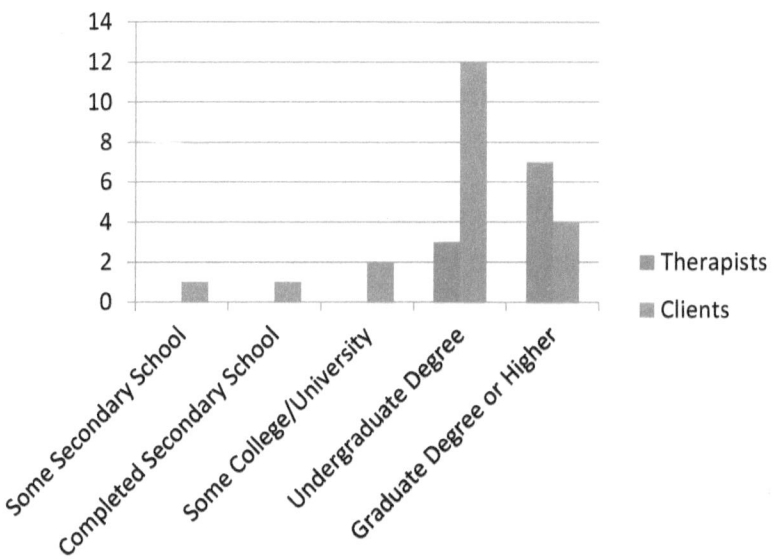

Figure 2.

Education

Percentage of Study Participants

This information suggested that the clients have a significantly high level of postsecondary education and that many of the participants are likely to be able to read and understand the approaches to therapy, the methods for discussing end-of-life meaning, and significant concepts related in the psychoanalytical praxis.

The client subject population, the population participating primarily in the survey and focus group elements, was all over the age of sixty-five. The mean age of the group was seventy-six years with the youngest participant sixty-eight years of age and the oldest participate ninety-two years of age. The participant group was overwhelmingly female, with fourteen of the twenty being female participants and six being male participants. The therapist group was significantly younger, with a mean age of fifty-four, and a larger group of male participants (three-fifths of the group male and two-fifths of the group female).

❧ Thematic Findings by Question

The thematic findings related to each of research questions and derived from multiple assessment approaches include information recorded during focus group and interview experiences. A thematic grouping approach was applied to the transcribed recordings in order to identify consistent themes and create a body of thematic information that can be understood in the context of the therapeutic relationships. Each research question was provided, and the thematic data was identified with quotes from participants in tables 1–6.

The first research question introduced and evaluated with thematic findings is this: What are the main characteristics of an effective therapist when addressing issues in end-of-life planning?

Table 1. The themes that emerged from an evaluation of the data collected include the desire for effective communication, frankness, and goal setting. The participants generally believe that the therapeutic relationship is beneficial and that to maintain that benefit, they must be willing to do the "hard work." Effective communication was a goal, but some of the statements made by the participants reflected difficulties in communicating effectively with therapists. For example, one individual maintained that he felt that the therapist did not always state what he meant, and there was sometimes confusion in their communications.

Table 1

Question 1: What are the main characteristics of an effective therapist when addressing issues in end-of-life planning?

Open Code	Properties	Example of Participant Words
Communication	Effective communication is identified as communication that addresses the needs of the client while also ensuring that messages are shared with clarity.	Negative: "doesn't say what he means" "not sure what he's asking" "doesn't address my issues" Positive: "talks about what I need to talk about" "knows I'm struggling and asks about it"
Frankness	Frankness reflects the ability of the therapist to share an honest appraisal of the situation or to talk about difficult subjects.	"gives it to me straight" "sometimes he knows I don't want to talk about things, but he pushes me" "reminds me why I'm here"
Goal Setting	Goal setting means sharing expectations about what will occur in the therapeutic interaction and how those goals will be reached.	"know where we're going each time" "communication is key" no room for therapist to be "wishy-washy"

The coding of comments made in the focus group also supported the belief that therapists should be effective in supporting goals setting and ensuring that communication is in alignment with client goals. Goal setting was described by one of the participants as an expectation of how they will interact and what will occur in the therapeutic setting. One of the participants stated that she felt the new praxis was beneficial in creating a more active communication with her therapist, who she had been seeing for five years.

The second research question introduced and evaluated with thematic findings is this: What are you looking for in therapy in terms of your fears, anxieties, or expectations? (table 2). The themes that emerged from an evaluation of the data collected include fear of death, anxiety, family issues, problems with end-of-life decision-making, loss of autonomy.

Table 2

Question 2: What are you looking for in therapy in terms of your fears, anxieties, or expectations?

Open Code	Properties	Example of Participant Words
Fear of death	Fear of death was identified as a major issue people sought to address in therapy. One subject described fear of death as "fear of the unknown."	"debilitating fear" "lack of control" "finality"

Anxiety	Anxiety was identified as an issue that was reflected in loss of sleep, loss of a desire to do normal things, and a loss of emotional ease.	"pressure to solve issues" "death is the end" "fear and anxiety" "shame over being afraid" "lacking faith in an afterlife"
Family issues	Subjects identified family problems with end-of-life care as an issue.	"involved in the decision-making process" "communications" "feeling part of a team"
End-of-life decision-making	End-of-life decision-making, including advanced directives and wills, was identified as an issue.	"share expectations" "positive feedback" "control"
Loss of autonomy	Two subjects discussed the issue of lost physical ability and the grief related to the lack of an ability to make personal decisions.	"involved in the decision-making process" "don't want to lose my faculties" "humiliation'

Question 2 sparked the largest amount of discussion of any of the questions and related the desire to explore a variety of issues involved in aging. Five of the participants mentioned loss of autonomy as a major issue that they wanted to explore in the therapeutic process. Two of the participants discussed issues of end-of-life decision-making, and two discussed the fact that family members were in dispute with them about end-of-life care issues. Family issues also resulted in descriptions of the ultimate family situation, in which family members would participate as a part of a care team and all members would be involved in decision-making.

The two commonly held reasons for pursuing an existential psychoanalytical approach were the development of death fear and death anxiety. Though participants did not use that specific verbiage, they did relate major issues with anxiety, including fear of the unknown and shame over their lack of faith in the afterlife, as significant indictors of the onset of anxiety. Four participants discussed the issue of fear in global terms related to the "end of life as we know it." These reflections suggest that the participants are actively discussing the need for methods to explore existential questions.

The third research question introduced and evaluated with thematic findings is this: Have you experienced any benefits from your therapist using the new existential praxis? (table 3). The themes that emerged from an evaluation of the data collected include level of experience, need for training, resistance, and motivation. Though it was not the intention of this question to foster a discussion about the limitations or resistance of therapists, this did come out as a natural progression of the data collection process. The participants maintained that while the therapists they worked with seemed willing to implement the new strategy, they were not fully able to explain it or to ensure that it was in alignment with the expectations of the researcher. One woman stated that her therapist worked with the praxis one day and then did not go back to it. This information was collected in narrative form and utilized to explain some of the outcomes in relation to questions about benefits of the approach.

Table 3

Question 3: Have you experienced any benefits from your therapist using the new existential praxis?

Open Code	Properties	Example of Participant Words
Level of experience	The greater the level of experience with the praxis was necessary in order to support, willingness of staff is to implement change.	"difference in the level of experience" "willingness to implement change" "therapist seemed unsure"
Need for training	Training is a tool that can improve reception to change.	practitioners seemed "unsure of process" and were more comfortable with their "traditional approach"

Resistance	Resistance to change occurs at all levels and can include resistance by therapist and resistance by client.	need to see "the connection … to results" "feedback" is helpful in reducing resistance
Motivation	Therapists need to be motivated to change.	"seems stuck in his ways" "doesn't want to use the new system"

The participants in the focus group stated that they could not see a connection between the process and the results that they hoped to achieve. Goal setting, they maintained, was an approach that could have been used in conjunction with the proposed praxis to ensure notable results.

The fourth research question introduced and evaluated with thematic findings is this: How effective is your therapist in providing the support you need to address concerns about end-of-life experiences? (table 4). Generally, the subjects noted that this was a difficult element and that they were generally happy with their experiences in the therapeutic setting. They did reflect on the belief that treatment is beneficial when it is in alignment with specific goals and that this ensures a connection between the role of the therapist and the role of the individual. At the same time, as viewed in table

4, at least six of the participants noted that they did not like some of the verbiage used in discussions about their process and therapeutic experiences, including terms like "end-of-life planning" and "elderly care needs."

Table 4

Question 4: How effective is your therapist in providing the support you need to address concerns about end-of-life experiences?

Open Code	Properties	Example of Participant Words
Different treatment	Distinct treatment is provided and has beneficial outcomes.	"need to continue" "beneficial outcomes related to goals"
Verbiage	The language used to discuss this kind of issue is not always conducive to positive discussions.	don't like "end-of-life planning" and "elderly care needs" "there are better ways to frame this information in the therapeutic relationship"

The fifth research question introduced and evaluated with thematic findings is this: Do you believe that your experiences in therapy have helped you address concerns you have about the meaningfulness of your life? (table 5). The themes that emerged from an evaluation of the data collected include the need for change and the brevity of life. These themes emerged in a number of forms, and the focus group became a group therapy session after that question was asked. Each time an individual made a statement, including things like "I'm a work in progress," their comments were followed by statements made by a number of other participants in support of what they said. A repeated theme by seven of the group participants was the idea of wanting to be remembered by others. In addition, the theme of the brevity of life was emphasized by two of the older participants in the group, who maintained that their lives seemed to have passed too quickly and they regretted not having taken advantage of opportunities when they were younger.

Table 5

Question 5: Do you believe that your experiences in therapy have helped you address concerns you have about the meaningfulness of your life?

Open Code	Properties	Example of Participant Words
Need for change	Individuals maintained that even as they age, they are constantly moving toward a state of self-improvement.	"I'm a work in progress" "I'm not sure I'll know if it's meaningful until it's over" "I want to be remembered"

Brevity of life	Life is short, and this complicates the issue of attaining meaningfulness.	"it has gone by too fast" "if I only knew what I know now when I was a kid, I wouldn't have wasted so much time"

The subjects were also asked to respond to a sixth research question, which was this: Can you discuss any improvements to the praxis that has been introduced? There were no significant comments about this element, so no thematic coding was utilized. The general comment made by just one participant was that most of them are happy to be a part of a therapy process that addresses their concerns specifically, so they "do not complain."

❋ Interview Questions

The interview questions covered much of the same information introduced in the focus group but were conducted of therapists to determine their perspectives on the existential psychoanalytical praxis and the implications for addressing client needs. The approaches that were related reflected the value of exploring issues of life, death fear, death anxiety, meaningfulness, and self-actualization. Figure 3 demonstrates what the therapists perceived as their capacity to improve patient outcomes over the course of a six-week treatment process. The participants were asked to specifically assess their views of the impacts of the praxis on death fear, death anxiety, and self-actualization.

Figure 3.

Success of the Praxis

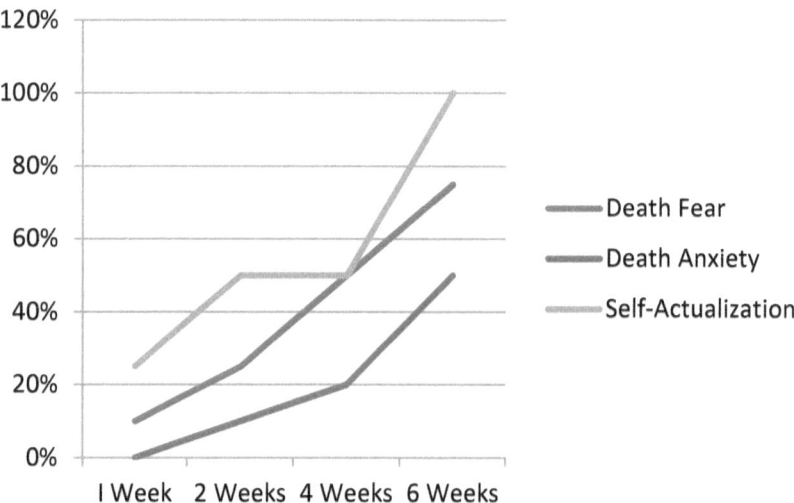

Figure 3 reflects the overall perceptions of success identified by the therapists and addressed some of the central perceptions related in the focus group, including the view of one of the subjects that her therapist only applied the praxis one time. Figure 4 provides a view of the therapists' perceptions of how much of the time during the therapeutic interaction they addressed the central elements that influence the existential process for the elderly, including death fear, death anxiety, and self-actualization. This figure demonstrates a rise over time in the number of opportunities to address these functional elements and suggests that practice with the praxis over time improves the ability to focus on central elements.

Figure 4.

Therapist Perceptions of Elements Addressed

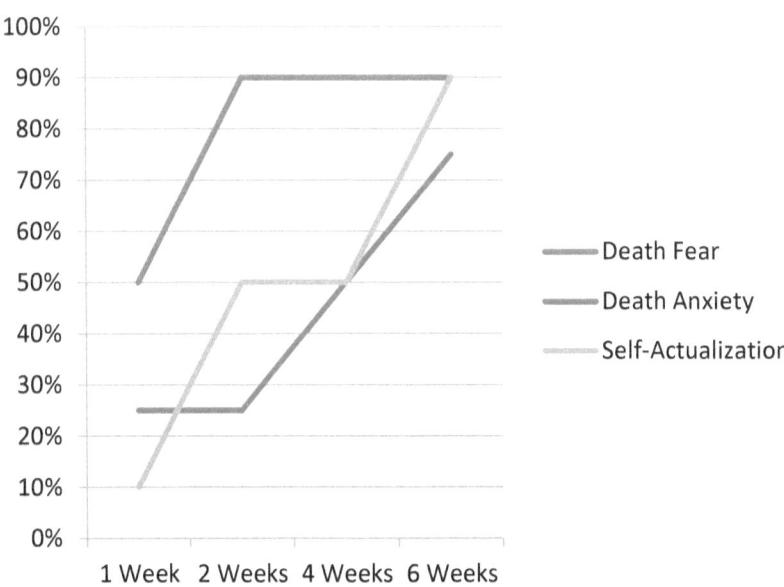

The data collected from interviews, the focus group, and survey materials for the therapists and clients at the facility reflect specific views of the approach, the ability to create a responsive relationship, and the ability to meet goals for addressing fundamental issues. The data reflects a division between the perspectives of some of the therapists on the best approaches to achieving goals and the varied views of clients about the success in applying the praxis to their therapeutic process. At the same time, the data also underscores perceived benefits of this approach, including addressing some of the functional identified issues in end-of-life experiences, including death fear, death anxiety, and self-actualization.

❇ Discussion

The research findings correspond with many of the views of the way in which therapeutic approaches are used to address the needs of aging populations. The existential praxis focuses on the role of the therapist or counselor in addressing the functional needs of the individual while also supporting an aim toward self-actualization. This corresponds with Rogers's 1946 view that traditional models often leave individuals responsible for any kind of therapeutic change by themselves. "The counselor [frequently] operates on the principle that the individual is basically responsible for himself, and is willing for the individual to keep that responsibility" (Rogers 415). The therapist does not detract from the client's own process or their skills toward change but supports the motivation toward wellness, which may dictate the need for change. This type of approach has been identified through its longevity and the continued application of phenomenological research. Mearns and Thorne maintained that many therapists or counselors have recognized the benefits of creating equality in a counseling relationship and that this equity has helped them support the work of clients in achieving self-actualization. The limitation of this perspective that is addressed through the existential paradigm though comes in relation to its application and to the issues that individuals bring to the relationship that can impact the communication between the therapist and individual.

Mearns and Thorne argued that while most therapists see the benefit of creating equity in their interactions with clients, they do not necessarily find it easy to maintain. In fact, these researchers have argued that it is more common for therapists to establish inequity as a component of the therapeutic relations. "The counselor is on familiar territory; the client is not." Subsequently, the counselors may find it difficult to ensure an empathetic and viable process through which the exploration of end-of-life issues can be ensured.

✖ The Stigma and Terror of Death

The research relating to the views of focus group participants and even some therapists indicate that one of the challenges that emerges when discussing the application of an existential paradigm to the therapeutic relationship for elderly patients is that there is such a range of views on the issue of death and dying. Irvin Yalom maintained that the issue of human mortality requires an existential perspective applied to a greater awareness of human function, consciousness, and the significance of death fear. Yalom actually defined the concept of death anxiety, maintaining that while death fear is an immediate and natural component of the process of life (e.g., animals experience fear responses in the presence of threats to life), death anxiety is a purely human response to the cultural, social, and psychological views of dying and death. Yalom described self-awareness as a "supreme gift" but also recognized that it comes with its share of costs (283), not the least of which is a constantly haunting sense of our own mortality.

For most people, fear of death enters our existence

periodically, usually in response to the death of loved one, a pet, a friend, a neighbor, or the presence of a national tragedy (e.g., 9/11). This may result in a sense of unrest or may be hidden and manifest in some masqueraded version through specific psychological symptoms, but death anxiety is a disruptive and complex process through which explicit thoughts of death dominate personal perspective. Death anxiety and terror can be so explicit in an individual's life that they can be disruptive to the process of daily functioning. Yalom recognized that as people age and the period of the end of life grows closer, the concept of death anxiety becomes more acutely recognizable and may become a prevalent component of daily experience.

While Yalom's perspective provides insight into the underlying causation of death fear and death anxiety, it does not essentially define the best approach to addressing these elements in reflection of the needs of an aging population. One of the reasons for this is that dying and death, though personal and individual processes, are elements in which society in general finds cause to constantly comment. Our culture defines the way we view death and the way we identify the mourning of lost opportunities that correspond with end-of-life experiences. The need to address death from a new existential psychoanalytical approach extends from the fact that is it no longer a simple act of the cessation of life but a source of existential angst that requires a principled view of the cultural manifestations of death, its stigma, and the implications for aging.

From a social perspective, life used to be the process by which we obtained personal fulfillment through the completion of life through a cyclical process of human development. Death then was simply the completion of that process, or the end of a cycle of life. While humans have always naturally feared death and seek methods of avoidance when possible, the end of death was not always perceived as a social objectionable result of the failure of a medical system, scientific process, or socially desirable whim. An oversimplification of the process now is that death is perceived as an enigmatic enemy that should be avoided through the application of technologies at any cost. Modern medicine has changed the view of death from a necessary element of the cycle to an institutionalized issue to be fought.

It's hard to determine which came first: the views of death as a demon to be avoided or the legal and ethical debates about end-of-life decision-making and the ethics of care for the elderly. When debating decisions that can be made near the end of life, legal, ethical, religious, and moral ideals come into play and determine how to clean up the process of death while making it inherently palatable to all of those involved as stakeholders. The medicalization of death and the views of the use of methods to create easy death have been controversial. Clearly, in defining the marginalization of dying, roles for family members have shifted from carative to decision-making. At the same time, while decisions about life and death can be made by family members at the request of medical professionals, legal parameters do not support decisions about death outside the structure of a hospital setting. Support for concepts like euthanasia in cases where individuals are in extreme pain, are severely ill, or are severely incapacitated has had significant support but only serves to detract from the importance of resolving the cultural conundrum of death.

Philosophical perspectives can be helpful in understanding the arguments of good actions and good intentions in determining the ethics of medical advancements to either increasing longevity or cause the cessation of life. There are two essential principles: the deontological principle and utilitarianism, both of which inform how to assess the actions of individuals seeking answers about choices in the presence of inevitable death.

The deontological principle is based on the belief

that if the actions of the individual are viewed as good, the action, regardless of its outcomes, is also good. If in the course of a situation, however, there is an inherent contradiction, one that brings into question the goodness of the action, the action itself is wrong. For example, the actions of the health care workers that resulted in the death of patients may have had a desirable end. The doctors and nurses may have maintained that the continuation of life would have resulted in the continuation of suffering, so they may have sought techniques to end life earlier. While the outcomes of this process may be perceived as inherently good, if just one family member questions the benefits of this process, the overall goodness of the action cannot be determined.

The deontological perspective then demonstrates that if there is a contradiction, if

> in the nature of action, a contradiction is found, then that is the rational evidence, the sufficient condition, to determine that the action is wrong. An appeal to good making consequences is neither necessary nor sufficient. (Roberts)

Subsequently, the actions of the nurses and doctors reflected poor decision-making and unethical behaviors that determined positive outcomes. From the deontological perspective, these actions are unethical and inherently problematic. From the most ethical and moral standpoint, the deontological approach is the most commonly applied in the modern society and has directed the debate regarding approaches to care and methods for negating support from specific actions when pursued at the end of life.

Utilitarianism is often applied to a view of choices, including the ethics and the behaviors of professionals faced with end-of-life care. John Stuart Mill maintained that many people act in a utilitarian manner, to seek "pleasure and freedom from pain" because these are the "only things desirable as ends" (Mill, as cited by Albanese 37). An action is perceived as utilitarian if it provides the greatest good for the greatest number of people. In the marginalization of death, the greatest good is perceived in relation to removing the view of death from human experience and creating "comfortable" ways of addressing the needs of the elderly. This detracts though from the authenticity of life and from the importance of methods to validate the process aging. Conway recognized that this has also resulted in the progression of ideals based on the legal and government control of death, rather than in creating authentic experiences linked back to Heidegger's conceptual view of being in the world and the authentic experience rationales offered by May, Maslow, and Rogers.

ⅸ Existential Questions and Aging

The oversimplification of what has been deemed the "problem of death" and the efforts to create an answer to the problem have led to the perception that as people age, they no longer need to ask the essential existential questions about meaning. This creates a considerable gap between those who are making medical, social, and practical decisions related to dying and death and those who are progressing through the life span. There is a clear necessity to create an understanding of the aging process and to identify and validate the progression of life and existential concerns of older people (Langle and Probst 193). An existential psychological approach alone does not fully address the foundational nature of these questions, the connection between culturally influenced perspectives on death and the individual development of death fear, or the connection between the disinvestment in authentic experiences of dying from a social or cultural standpoint and the development of death anxiety in response to existential concerns.

Langle and Probst recognized that existential questioning for the elderly raises specific issues that can be influenced by a range of factors, including the transitory nature of life itself, the coping mechanisms that an individual develops over the life span, and the impacts of enduring illness and suffering. In addition, researchers and theorists, including Allport (284), Feifel and Nagy (278), and Delongis and Holtzman (166), recognized that a range of components feed into the sense of self that shapes a person's need for assessing self-worth at the end of life. Actual views on life and death and beliefs about the importance of meaningfulness are deeply ingrained in the progression of self-identity that relates to a lifetime of experiences. Correspondingly, responses to life experiences, stressors, anxiety-provoking thoughts of life and death, and significant life changes all hinge on the coping mechanism and social support factors that are obtained and progress over the life span (Delongis and Holtzman 166).

For some, old age is simply the sum total of experiences and individuals are capable of confronting existential questions about the meaning of life based on some of their long-standing coping mechanisms. For example,

Langle and Probst (193) recognized that older adults who have religious beliefs that drive their daily life are more apt to identify religious purpose as a factor in determining their approach to both living and dying. The conceptual view of the will of a higher power is often a comforting thought that also serves to reduce anxiety and depression in end-of-life experiences (Langle and Probst 193). At the same time, the will of a higher power can also be what drives individuals to continue life in the presence of pain and suffering, and it certainly has specific implications for political, social, and cultural debates on end-of-life decisions.

Older adults also experience conflicts related to the very real experiences of their lives at a time when mortality becomes increasingly evident. Older adults not only face their own mortality but also the mortality of family members, loved ones, and social contacts. Evidence mounts for older adults about the transitory nature of life, the need to identify purpose, and the ability to place meaning on both life and death (Langle and Probst 195). One eighty-two-year-old woman in the study told the story of the systematic death of each person she had known since childhood. First she related the fact that her parents died when she was in her sixties, both her best friend since childhood and her husband of fifty-three years in her seventies, and then twelve members of her church in the last five years. Then she described the fact that she felt increasing loneliness and identified a purpose for death: so she would no longer be alone. Though loneliness in the elderly population is a contributory factor for depression, this woman did not see herself as depressed. Instead, she maintained that she had a very pragmatic view on her life and stated that she simply never imagined she would outlive everyone in her social circle. "I guess someone had to."

This kind of perspective provides some insight into the complicated nature of addressing the psychological and psychosocial needs of aging adults and the issues that also extend from applying psychiatric, psychological, or psychoanalytical models that do not incorporate an existential element to the experiences of this population. Evaluations of the eighty-four-year-old subject might have resulted in the assessment that she is depressed and/ or has a significant level of death anxiety. Depending on the breadth of symptoms that she demonstrates in an evaluation setting, she might also be experiencing elements of posttraumatic stress disorder following the death of so many family members and friends. All of these things do not place her experiences, frame of references, or even her own admitted pragmatism into an equation to address her process of dying and death. "Managing" the problems related to end-of-life care, including loneliness, anxiety, and depression, becomes the focal point of treatment paradigms instead of methods to see past these elements toward a greater understanding of the purposeful nature of dying.

Langle and Probst described death as "one of the big tasks of man" and related two approaches that are generally taken to address this process: examination/exploration of the process or a stagnant suppression/sequestration. In addition to these two separate and distinctly difference approaches, old age is something that the elderly are experiencing in isolation of the world, rather than as members of it. The elderly experience the physical loss of loved ones at the same time that they are sent away to live with others who are aging, who have lost their mental capabilities, or who can no longer live autonomously due to physical illness or injury. "Forced to silence without anything to say because you are not asked any more leads to dissolution of important relationships in life." The connections of social structure that support a running commentary on the importance of life become the same connections attempting to quell the voice of those who are moving toward death. Discourse on death can be uncomfortable, disheartening, depressing, and without a workable solution, so those who participate in the discourse from a position of anticipation are marginalized. "Thus old age powerfully pushes man back into himself" (Langle and Probst 196).

An existential perspective provides a foundation for recognizing some of the uncomfortable truths about life and death that need to be addressed in the process of growing old. Specifically, that life is not without pain, that human existence and the progression toward death is a natural component of the life cycle, and that personal autonomy is often derived from an understanding of what life means in the process of dying. The existential questions of meaning, purpose, spirituality, and loss of presence in the world become central in the minds of the aging, while they are frequently ignored until a person faces death (Malette and Oliver 30).

One of the interesting revelations in regard to the exploration of psychological theories and foundational elements for addressing aging and end-of-life process is that perspectives on aging and death appear to be coming in full circle. More than a half century ago, theorists like Birren (1) and Butler (8) introduced studies about the importance of developing an experiential perspective on death, one that was highly personalized and reflected the importance of deriving meaning from life. Unfortunately, this kind of existential psychological perspective fell out of favor for more highly mechanized views on mental health and solution-focused approaches to death. Though existential principles could be applied to gaining meaning about the purpose of life or avenues for personal growth at a variety of points during the life span, they stopped being applied to the progression of the aging identity in the presence of the unanswerable problem of death. Death suddenly became an issue to be avoided, and elderly individuals struggling with existential angst were pushed to seek the support of antidepressants rather than explore their existential questions.

An existential psychoanalytical approach that addresses some of the foundational issues for the elderly, while also exploring answers to questions of purpose and meaning, can be supported by the assertions of authors like Langle and Probst, who argued that existential challenges inherent appear in this process that require the redefinition of "one's being-in-the-world by attributing meanings to the joys, accomplishments, and losses of one's life." This also includes determining potential threats to the dignity of an aging individual, relating what that person perceives as culturally directed quests to address that threat, the identification of existential needs in life, and the use of a psychoanalytical process to determine resolution.

Birren described this in relation to both the psychological influences impacting individuals as they age and the mesh of elements that combine to form experiential views of life's meaning and purpose. Birren described this as the "fabric of life," while Butler maintained the importance of continually revisiting the history of life and recognizing it is influence on the process of "successful aging."

❇ The Identification and Purpose of the Praxis

Existential psychoanalysis requires more than just an understanding of potential answers to foundational questions; it also requires an understanding the impacts of socially and culturally defined experiences in the past on end-of-life activities to answer existential questions. This includes acceptance of some of the principle aspects of the existential angst: that humans have both the animalistic drive for survival and the need to accept death as a component of life (Lee 303). This kind of view relates the very personal nature of experiences related to both life and death and the need to consider the implications for an individualized therapeutic process (Cooper 87, 2005). The complication that arises in applying either a traditional approach to psychoanalysis or a more fluid humanistic or existential approach is that both of these methods have limitations in meeting the transformational needs of an aging person nearing the end of life (Choron 88).

This perspective is shaped by the view that a person may have many different experiences influencing their perceptions of the meaning of death through the course of their lifetime. One of the subjects, a seventy-two-year-old man, had a range of perspective related to his interpretation of death and said in the past he had "a much easier time of it." He stated that he was a war veteran and there was a time when he was able to take the lives of others without a thought. "You just did it." As he began to face his own aging and the reality of his own mortality, he found himself reflecting on each life he had taken in war and wondered how many of them debated "the end before it happened." The evolutionary nature of these kinds of reflections and the views of individuals that change during the life span are clearly components of the therapeutic interaction that need to be addressed to contextualize end-of-life process (Whelton 156; Trust et al., 66).

The existential praxis provides a means of understanding the differentiated experiential views influencing the response to specific questions. This can include the variety of elements that impact perceptions of death as well as experiences that shape a person's response to the immediacy of death. For example, the social context or spiritual belief systems of an individual can be helpful in responding to questions like "What happens after death?" The insecurity that a person feels in the presence of this question might be answered when applying a religious perspective.

For those without this kind of foundational belief system, an existential psychoanalytical praxis can provide a means of addressing both the factors in life influencing perceptions of end-of-life issues and the context in which those factors developed. In many cases, individuals attempt to address the shift in their views on existential purpose, meaning, and death experiences. In the past, elderly were valued, rather than marginalized, and death was a sequential component of life (Birren 3). The medicalization of the process of dying and modernization of medical technologies have led to the creation of many different conundrums surrounding the issue of death that create an intellectualized view of death as an essential problem in modern society (Lee 291; Walter 293). This leads to the need for an approach to psychoanalysis for elderly adults that takes into account the varied perspectives on death and the changing societal, cultural, and spiritual views of dying and death.

Walter, for example, maintained that dying and death

are the antithesis of the elements valued in modern society: youth and health. As the elderly move closer and closer to death, they become "uniquely isolated, lepers even, because they highlight the Achilles heel of the modern individual." They are marginalized because they represent a threat to the values of the modern society and their very existence brings into question the ability of individuals to maintain their own youth. Though there are many who are not aging who have physical impairments or illnesses that challenge the perfection of youth and health, aging is differentiated from illness because illness can be shifted to the pursuit of wellness, while the elderly are irretrievably moving toward the end of their lives (McNamara 66). This defines a strange process for people going through what should be a normal and essential part of life. "Where postmodern dying finds us bereft of ways to approach death as a collective, medicalized dying pushes the phenomenon of death away through technology and presence."

Walter maintained that the lack of spiritual support around the process of death further supported the ritualization of death, the medicalization of death, and the creation of death taboo, defined by the belief that death should be medically preventable. The belief that the failure of the medical system leads to death, rather than the view of the inevitability of death, has led to increased death fear. The existential questions surrounding life and death and the integration of those questions into a sometimes conflicted societal context of death is the underlying purpose of the existential psychoanalytical praxis.

The contextualization of experience related to the sense of self-actualization relates the process of psychological development to principles of self-actualization linked to Heidegger's philosophy and Rogers's therapeutic approach. It also provides a focus for the development of a feasible existential psychoanalytic process, which takes into consideration the views of May, Maslow, and Rogers but also integrates the philosophical approaches to identifying self-value. The conflicted views of death are inextricably linked to perceptions regarding the value placed on life. Subsequently, while life should be valued at all costs, death, which is a natural component of the progression of life, is societal taboo.

❧ Summary

The existential psychoanalytic praxis requires an assessment of the factors within the modern society that define the value placed on both the self-actualized life and the process of dying and death, specifically reflecting upon the problematic nature of death. Death is perceived as a weakening and a dark element that shadows the self-actualized life. Any contributory factors to the progression of death, whether they are pain, suffering, or bereavement for the loss of others, feed into the designed taboo. Efforts to legitimize death as a part of life frequently look to the spiritual elements, which do not truly legitimize death but simply view it as a spiritual vehicle by which the individual soul moves on to the afterlife. The data presented underscores the importance of evaluating the specific factors and existential questions the elderly face while also assessing perceptions of the benefits of a new approach to psychoanalysis. This praxis is rooted in the contextualization of death views and the identification of existential questions as a component of the psychoanalytical process.

CHAPTER 5
IMPLICATIONS AND RECOMMENDATIONS

Necessity of the Dissertation

ESSENTIALLY, VIEWS ON DYING AND DEATH have been transformed by social and cultural shifts over the last half century. At the same time that technological changes have led to the growth of the elderly population in this country, questions about mortality, the limitations of human life, and its meaning have been placed on the back burner. Subsequently, the elderly have been encouraged to fight death and to deny the presence of death fear, death anxiety, and existential questions. Even the terminology utilized in health care and medical literature about longevity, medical responses, and medical capabilities refer to vague concepts like medical futility and ethical decision-making in end-of-life care that rationalize or intellectualize the problem of death (Curtis and Burt 1742; Haynes 36; Schneiderman 123). In many cases, the pursuit of any reflective process by which individuals explore the issue of death is viewed as negative, and health technology is asserted as the solution to the medical problem of death (Battin 7; Butts and Rich 270; Casper 11; Lehoux 2). Existential views have been related as a means of grounding some of the broader perspectives on the transformation of the modern culture and the sequestration of death by way of creating solutions to death as a problem (Farber 289).

The creation of an existential psychoanalytical praxis that addressees the specific needs of the elderly is clearly a novel process that relates the difference between the meaning of death for the elderly and the meaning of death for those facing terminal illnesses at another time in life. This praxis includes a focus on the threats to dignity, the culturally directed quests that may be differentiated from seeking meaning or defining existential purpose, the existential life needs of the elderly, and the methods to resolve the gap between culturally directed ideals and existential needs through an existential psychoanalytical process. (See appendix.) At a time when there is a growing elderly population in the United States and continued social and cultural sequestration of death, this approach poses a method of addressing the needs of the elderly.

⅜ New Conceptual View

The exploration of themes and literature related to the transformation of views of death for elderly populations led to the identification of a goal of the therapeutic process: successful aging.

The identification of the concept of successful aging in the course of exploring the research was a surprising element that emerged in attempting to define existential goals (Butler 529). One of the most interesting elements that came out in relating past and present views on the elderly, their perspectives, and the views of therapists is that there was a method of successfully achieving end goals for elderly clients who were in the end period of their life: to successfully navigate issues related to death fear, death anxiety, and questions of meaningfulness through the pursuit of a state of self-actualization.

Both Maslow and Rogers recognized the importance of self-actualization in the pursuit of a greater sense of meaning in life and explored a range of elements, including spirituality and self-worth, as a means of achieving self-actualization. Maslow, for example, maintained that people who have serious psychological issues benefitted from the exploration of existential questions in order to develop a coherent sense of self and to support optimal functioning. Self-actualized people then were able to identify reality, recognize the parameters of reality within a social context, and create a clear sense of themselves within this context. Self-actualized individuals were independent and private and bring their own sense of self to their social culture. Maslow maintained that self-actualized people shared the following qualities:

- truth rather than dishonesty
- goodness rather than evil
- beauty rather than ugliness
- utility, wholeness, and transcendence of opposites, not arbitrariness or forced choices
- aliveness, not deadness or the mechanization of life
- uniqueness, not bland uniformity
- perfection and necessity, not sloppiness, inconsistency, or accident
- completion, rather than incompleteness
- justice and order, not injustice and lawlessness
- simplicity, not unnecessary complexity
- richness, not environmental impoverishment

- effortlessness, not strain
- meaningfulness rather tha senselessness

The ideal approach to supporting the elderly during the end-of-life period is to implement an existential psychoanalytic approach that focuses on steps based on self-actualization goals while also ensuring recognition of the factors and processes defined by changing views on death. The connection between self-actualization and the creation of a successful aging process aligns this developed theoretical perspective to the praxis described.

❊ Ideal Existential Psychoanalytic Approach for End of Life

The ideal existential psychoanalytic approach to the exploration of successful aging, or the end-of-life process, is an amalgamation of existing approaches. It is rooted in some of the foundational views of May, Maslow, and Rogers and then considers the functional factors and progression of identifying characteristics that define experiences around the process of dying and death. In order to successfully achieve a process of discourse that is valuable to ensuring self-actualization (a goal related to successful aging), the praxis supports a humanistic view of the influences on self-identification and supports a cultural view of the defining and redefining of death.

One of the struggles in creating this kind of an approach is that views on aging and death have changed significantly in recent decades. Rituals surrounding death are created to foster the sequestration of death and work to define death as a resoundingly difficult social problem. Death appears not as a final bow at the end of a successful performance of life but as a weakening decline that devalues much of what comes before it in life. The anticipation of death brings with it culturally defined values about the belief that death is a problem that could not be resolved. From medical, social, and even spiritual beliefs, death is problematic and reflects failure to find a solution (Mellor and Shilling 427). Legitimization of death as an actual component of life is a necessary part of the existential psychoanalytic process, supporting the inevitability of death and greater awareness of the importance of death in acknowledging the value of life.

Another significant challenge in developing an existential psychoanalytic praxis is recognizing that there are distinct variables that impact how individuals perceive the progression of their lives. For example, if a person is spiritual and believes in an afterlife in heaven, they may feel either relief at the idea of death or shame over their fear. As one of the focus group participants noted, if a person had a developed and faithful religious life, they would not fear death. At the same time, there are differences in the way religious or spiritual beliefs are applied to the conceptualization of death. If a person believes that their spirit leaves this world and goes on to the afterlife in heaven, never to return, the gap widens between the known and the unknown. This can be fear provoking even for those who have a very ingrained religious perspective. If, however, a person's spiritual beliefs incorporate reincarnation, the idea that the person may return in a different form over and over again may provide comfort and reduce the belief that death is a negative. Death, as one subject noted in their interview, could be seen as just a step along the path of greater self-actualization.

One of the major contributing elements to this praxis though is Rogers's belief that self-actualization is a significant component of any therapeutic process. Successful movement in this type of relationship requires an acceptance of basic elements, including the use of strategies to encourage conversation about issues like death and dying (Kirschenbaum 116). Rogers though sought to apply a nondirective method and to totally avoid questions, interpretations, suggestions, advice, and other direct techniques. Rather, it relied exclusively on a process of carefully listening to the client, accepting the client for who he or she is ... and skillfully reflecting back the client's feelings. (Kirschenbaum 116)

This approach suggests the use of facilitation approaches to support self-actualization but does not reflect the need for a phenomenological view of how individuals developed their insights about dying and death.

In the psychoanalytic praxis, the assessment of individual experiences and the contextualization of those experiences in relation to identifying characteristics of death is the largest component of the interaction between individual and therapist. The foundations of this approach link the identification of dysfunctional thoughts and processes to the significant actions or experiences, but this also has to reflect the fact that no one has experienced death fully before they die. Subsequently, the individual and therapist have to explore experiences related to self-perception, values, spirituality, culture, and self-actualization in order to relate their own perspective to the existential questions.

The phenomenological component of the existential praxis relates to both the experiences of the individual and the experience within the social culture and posits the belief that in an environment free of value judgments in which a person can explore fear, anxiety, shame, and other factors diminishing self-actualization, the aging adult can support the ability to obtain successful aging or aging toward self-actualization that ends in death. The role of the therapist in this process of successful aging then is to support the individual in "sensing meanings of which he or she is scarcely aware," which can include "communicating your sensings of the person's world" (Rogers). Subsequently, the repeated finding that communication and feedback are important elements of this dynamic model is indicated both by the perspectives of Rogers and the identification of unity, wholeness, and uniqueness as communicated by Maslow (Boeree 3). In addition, Maslow's belief in the perfection of the process and in the importance of completeness in the achievement of self-actualization are realized within the praxis an identification of existential life needs, an assessment of culturally directed quests, and the completion of the goals that are resolved through the existential approach.

The praxis can be applied to assessing the link between threats to dignity, culturally directed quests, and existential needs and provides an important method of assessing a range of issues, including death fear, death anxiety, guilt, or shame, helplessness, and anger, among many. For each of these, the praxis outlined as an example in the appendix demonstrates the connection between the threat and the quests that are applied by society and define expectations. For example, one of the reported elements regarding death fear that comes into play in the experiences individuals in the focus group is that most feel that they should fight against death, because out culture defines the need for protection from death. Death is the thing to be avoided at all costs. The existential perspective is that individuals have the capacity and courage for self-protection and that death in itself is not something from which we must inherently protect ourselves. The resolution through an existential psychoanalytic process would be based on an evaluation of feelings about death, feelings about the sequestration of death, and feelings about attempts to medically protect ourselves from death. The end product of this exploration, for example, could be the acceptance of death and the acknowledgment that death fear is about fear of the unknown.

Death anxiety, as defined within the scope of existing literature, is a set of physiological and psychological responses to the presence of "personal need to survive, to preserve our being, and to assert our being" (May and Yalom 3). Death anxiety is contrasted with normal anxiety that is proportional with the events that are occurring and does not create a physiological response or destructive life choices. Death anxiety then is a threat to dignity in aging that reflects some of the functional concerns about the shift in life and the need to be remembered, valued, and honored. The culturally directed quests in relation to death anxiety then become things like the reported need by some of the focus group and interview participants to be honored for what was accomplished in life as a means of reducing the feeling of meaningless in death. From an existential perspective, Rogers would maintain that the best response to death anxiety is the courage to pursue self-actualization, or as has been identified in this study as a new framing, the success of aging. The end product of a resolution process designed in the existential praxis would be the relief that occurs as a result of nonengagement in the discourse related to the sequestration of death.

Self-actualization can also come into play as an existential process at the end of life related to how a person perceives their abilities and their shortcomings. A threat to dignity related to self-actualization can be guilt or shame over the lack of perfection in life as life draws to a close. This is shaped by a culturally directed quest to achieve and the existential life need of courage to obtain freedom from imperfection and insecurity. A part of self-actualization that is important to successful aging in this area is the ability to apply self-forgiveness.

Despair is a commonly reported threat to dignity that was identified by a number of the subjects in the study, who argued it was linked to a sense that there is nothing better to come. This is impacted by the culturally directed quest for safety and freedom from pain and the conflicted realization that many things involving aging result in pain. The existential life needs that are the focus of the praxis would be to develop the courage to anticipate the meaning of the actions of others, especially in promoting autonomy and communication in end-of-life planning. This can lead to the resolution of hope through the existential psychoanalytic process, but hope seems a temporal outcome. In truth, hope does not embrace time parameters, so movement from despair to hope can be seen as a part of the process of self-actualization toward aging successfully.

Another threat to dignity in aging that can be a barrier to aging success is helplessness, both in physiological and psychosocial functioning. The culturally directed quest is one in which individuals are first identified as autonomous and valued for this and then are expected to relinquish their autonomy by giving up their decision-making to others. The existential life needs that can be applied to pursuing an understanding of these elements are the exploration of courage in seeking the support of others. This question speaks to the root of our life as an animal and as a part of a social collective. The capacity to explore this can result in addressing past issues that have impacted function and past problems that diminish the capacity for interactions with others. Truth and belief in others are the resolution.

Loss of self-worth is a threat to dignity that can be matched with both culturally directed quests and existential needs through the application of the praxis. In essence, loss of self-worth diminishes an individual's ability to see self-actualization as an achievable process. Loss of self-worth is defined by a culturally directed quest to be valued in the eyes of other people. The existential life needs include the courage to value self and the courage to accept self-actualization as the realistic end goals of life. The existential outcome is value, including value in both life and death, and value through self-actualization.

Anger is another threat to dignity that can benefit applying the existential praxis and developing a focus beyond the simple acts of anger relative to aging. One of the common feelings in the aging process is that there are many different things to be angry about. Loneliness can cause anger, as can the self of a loss of community and loved ones. Anger can stem from frustration or disbelief about the nature of life in the aging process. The culturally directed quests that often feed this include the belief that individuals always have a natural outlet for aggression that does not require identification of how the anger developed or progressed. The existential life need identified is the courage to transform experiences through an explorative process. The end product of anger then can be to experience joy based on the redefinition of elements and new experiences in alignment with these definitions. For example, the redefining of aging success can result in the belief that the same kinds of issues that were anger provoking can also be the fuel for experiencing joy.

Anxiety is an element that has to be taken into consideration in the application of the praxis and in creating a communicative relationship between therapist and client. Anxiety can be based on the creation of tension that can emerge from or exist prior to the onset of a therapeutic relationship. Anxiety continues in the presence of an attempt to create therapeutic congruence, as described by Rogers, because of the presence of a range of factors that are individualized and can influence process. Again, Rogers maintained that anxiety often emerges when there is a discrepancy between what a person views as their self-concept and areas in which change is necessary.

The concept of trust and the creation of a safe environment in which the client and therapist work on a common set of goals and a mechanism for the therapeutic process (Trusty, Ng, and Watts 66). This kind of process is indicative of the focus on the therapeutic relationship that is based on promoting the mental wellness of the client, but this is not always as easy as it sounds. In fact, finding a connection between elderly clients and their therapists can sometimes require a scrutinization of cultural elements that influence the development of views of the aging population.

Rogers believed in an interaction in which the "counselor operates on the principle that the individual is basically responsible for himself, and is willing for the individual to keep that responsibility." The therapist does not detract from the client's own process or their skills toward change but supports the motivation toward wellness, which may dictate the need for change.

Greenberg and Geller also maintained that some of these views of process were much more easily discussed as a theory than applied in the therapeutic relationship. In fact, these researchers maintained that out of the three basic conditions necessary for the therapeutic process (e.g., congruence, empathy, and unconditional positive regard), congruence was the most difficult for therapists to actually realize (Greenberg and Geller 150–151). Because there is a link between individual beliefs, intentions, and their applications to the roles of the therapist and client, the lack of awareness of their impact can inhibit the creation of effective communication, collaboration, or congruence.

Rogers and Sanford (1374) recognized that there are other conditions that can impact the relationship but supported the continued contention that communication is one of the skills that must be fine-tuned in order to achieve the necessary interaction with the client. Greenberg and Geller subsequently argued that this kind of focus can exist as the "most troublesome" of all the other conditions to realize, especially in cases where the client and therapist do not share common understanding, experiences, feelings, or needs. Whelton and Greenberg further maintained that a therapeutic approach may be limited by the fact that there is an inevitable level of subjectivity that can be applied to an understanding of the relationship and to the shaping of realities that can influence how a client perceives the interactions. These authors maintained that factors like attention, awareness, and the historical or experiential focus on learned experiences can shape the way in which progress in the therapeutic relationship is perceived.

❊ Recommendations

For older populations, it important to address factors that influence their perception of self and their capacity for change. As was noted by participants in the focus group and interviews, change can be a difficult thing, and people demonstrate resistance to change, whether a therapist implemented a new praxis or a patient using new techniques to explore views of death. A recommendation for future research could be to assess the role that therapists' views on a change initiative have for the implementation of new approaches for working with the elderly.

Another area of extended research has to do with the issue of communication. Many of the participants noted communication as an essential part of their response to the views of the therapists, especially when implementing a new praxis. This comes into play when considering the feasibility of implementing the new praxis. Evaluating some of the issues identified by elderly patients and creating a view of communication could be valuable in determining the best method for improving client outcomes.

Rodin maintained that relational decisions are often made that can either foster engagement or result in nonengagement, based on an evaluation of the benefits and costs of an interaction. Individuals frequently make choices about nonengagement based on their immediate responses, including their dislike of characteristics or their belief that the costs of interaction outweigh the benefits. This is especially true of people who are guarded or who may have a history of difficult communications. Older adults may find communications challenging and may find characteristics that result in nonengagement in the therapeutic environment. Approaches to create effective communication are important because they reduce the chances of "lapsed opportunities" that are based on the fear that receptivity would not exist and the belief that the costs were too high.

More than half of the focus group participants who actually participated in the discussion maintained that communication in the therapeutic environment was an element they perceived as supporting communication to resolve existential issues, especially when family members were involved. This kind of interaction can be based on fundamental beliefs about comfort and trust. Pearce maintained that there are three criteria that are necessary for trust: contingency, predictability, and options. Pearce further argued that necessity for knowledge, competence, and motivation in order to produce trusting behaviors that increase a person's vulnerability to the other person in the relationship and ensure a balance between both sides.

One of the frequent conflicts that have emerged in our modern culture is that trust does not always appear to be present in communications, or at least there are times when trust seems to be impacted by external factors, including cultural viewpoints and a lack of predictability. Pearce recognized that creating trust was based on a level of openness that created vulnerability. In interactions in this study, some of the resistance that emerged was based on both the desire to maintain a position of strength in the therapeutic relationship and the lack of a desire to earnestly address the problems many of the participants faced. In an interview, one of the participants identified feeling disquieted by holding a vulnerable posture, so deceit can be used as a tool to maintain disequilibrium that maintain a power structure. These elements come into play regardless of the praxis and can hinder the therapeutic experience. Subsequently, identifying these issues and the role they play in perceptions of the psychodynamic interaction can be important in assessing the selected praxis over time.

It is interesting to note that even in communications and interactions that are based on a therapeutic relationship, specific conflicts can emerge that pit the perspective of the therapist against the perspective of the client. This occurred in regard to the application of the selected praxis and the belief reiterated by one of the participants that her therapist refused to implement the praxis. Generally, conflicts emerged when a miscommunication occurred (e.g., which approach to use) that resulted in a lack of connection or when disagreements occur on a principal matter (e.g., refusal to participate). These conflicts were simply addressed by balancing the interests of the participants to the conflict at hand and the creation of plausible solutions. Avoidance techniques are sometimes utilized in order to address distress over conflict, and this appeared to happen in at least one of the therapeutic relationships.

This view goes back to the need to assess the Rogerian principles of the regard complex and the belief that self-experiences and interactions can have an influence on the therapeutic outcome. Rogers believed that there is a range of social elements that can influence the psychotherapeutic process and that the social connection can define how individuals respond to the process. Seeking methods to achieve self-actualization requires the exploration of self-experiences, which are symbolized and related in terms of self-concept. Subsequently, the communication element is essential to the effectiveness of this type of therapeutic praxis.

The exploration of the interaction between client and therapist through the application of both an existential approach and the psychoanalytical structure defines a distinct approach, but the aim is similar to that identified by Rogers. Rogers believed that the achievement of a fully functioning person was truly important and determined the need to develop interactions to foster this process through congruence. Rogers maintained that there are factors that include anxiety, threat, and disorganization that play a significant role in defining how individuals approach understanding of self. Subsequently, these were integrated in varying degrees into the assessment of the praxis because they provided a means of understanding discrepancies between desired status and the level of functioning present at the onset of therapy. Subsequently, some of these elements, including disorganization, can become a greater focus of research into the application of the praxis.

Greenberg and Geller maintained that cross-cultural perspectives may be beneficial in relating the role of the therapist and in distinguishing different factors that impact the therapeutic relationship.

> In our view it is always necessary for the therapist to be aware of her own feelings and reactions as this awareness orients her, and helps her be interpersonally clear and trustworthy. This inner awareness and contact naturally flows from the experience of therapeutic presence. (Greenberg and Geller 151)

The influence of culture on therapeutic presence should be considered in relation to the application of the praxis and in the capacity for bringing together the therapist and client in a common set of goals (Kirschenbaum 116).

An additional recommendation for future research is the assessment of cultural factors on the creation of a distinct definition of self-actualization. Repeatedly in the course of this study, references were made to Rogers's views of self-actualization and a greater body of the research hinged on this perspective. Self-actualization from Maslow's perspective incorporates a slightly different set of ideals, and it would be beneficial to consider the cultural influences that shape the concept. Depending on the approach and the methods, the different views on self-actualization can be beneficial. For example, both Rogers and Maslow share the importance of truth, unity, or wholeness, uniqueness, and meaningfulness as existential components of self-actualization. Maslow though added paired views of what constituted self-actualization that were not inherently identified in the views of Rogers. These include goodness rather than evil and aliveness rather than "not deadeness or the mechanization of life" (Boeree 3). In the creation of the existential praxis, the view of aliveness is not a necessity of the self-actualized individual, at least in terms of the views of how it can be applied to the exploration of existential angst related to death. Some of the participants in the focus group recognized that one of their struggles is that they may become the best example of themselves just before they have to leave this world.

Creating a concept analysis of self-actualization as the foundation for a study on its application would be a beneficial step in the research process. Though Maslow and Rogers provide a substantive body of information about the process of self-actualization, there is a range of views that can be incorporated and could include elements like social and spiritual self-actualization, which might be very different from the general frame of reference.

In assessing every aspect of personal development, it is important to consider how this information is fueled by social context, community, family, and religious views on the actions of aging adults.

✕ Implications

The research presented offers a novel approach that is the culmination of multiple views on existential process and on the application of a psychoanalytic structure to explore questions of life, meaning, and death. A key aspect of this is to ensure that aging adults can explore questions of their own mortality and address death fear and death anxiety while also recognizing cultural factors that influence their perceptions. This is all linked to major shifts in the way in which individuals are perceived and how their lives play out in relation to life, health, aging, and impending death. Though considerable efforts have been made to solve the problem of death, death continues to happen every day and is a reality for every person.

About a half century ago, the focus of the medical community was on the process of saving lives. The directive embraced by most medical professionals was not only "do no harm" but also "do everything that can be done." At the time, medical technology was burgeoning and the first thoughts of technology advancing past utility emerged in the form of the earliest forms of advanced directive or living will legislation in the 1970s. This was the first glimpse at the problem that would emerge from a zealous research community and the desire to advance medical technologies: the issue of whether individuals should live past their ability to sustain their own lives. The subsequent questions that emerged, including how these changes would change perceptions of death and how this would impact the psychological functioning of the elderly, were a part of the slow progression toward a problem-solving model for death.

Less than a half century later, advanced directives, living wills, and do-not-resuscitate orders are recognized documents that apply the perspectives of the elderly on the use of life-prolonging technologies. While it has been accepted that aging individuals can exert autonomy by utilizing these documents to demonstrate their will or decision-making in the absence of their ability to communicate those decisions, a different perspective has emerged in the care for the elderly: what if individuals want to simply age and die. Clearly, the existing literature and reflections of elderly adults participating in the therapeutic environment view conflicts, challenges, fear, and anxiety related to changing views of death.

In attempting to determine the best route to improve therapeutic interactions with an aging population and increase awareness of the issues facing the elderly, it is important to consider the demonization of illness and death and the application of a problem-solving approach. Most recently, researchers have maintained that the foundation of culture-driven policies in medical facilities has been to create a response to death that holds it at bay as long as possible. The concept of medical futility came out of the belief that some discourse had to be introduced to determine when medical interventions were no longer viewed as beneficial and when decision-makers should no longer seek to maintain life at all costs. This kind of approach has resulted in a clear shift from support for the progression of individuals through the life span to the introduction of methods to keep people alive in a manner that devalues the process of dying.

It is clear that debates on the issue of futility have led to questions about the way in which people live and die and how they are valued in relation to youth and health. Medical futility is often discussed in relation to the balance between medical treatment and the reality of human mortality; in every human life, there is a time at which the pursuit of life is no longer either medically prudent or in the best interest of the patient. Schneiderman maintained that when treatments can no longer result in a person being autonomous, the termination of medical services is viewed as an ethically sound choice. Further, even in the presence of life-sustaining technologies, decisions sometimes have to be made that "enough is enough."

The issue of medical futility has not only brought up discussions about mortality and the nature of medical interventions but also how people are valued and how death is perceived as a problematic component of treatment process. Death is inherently the failure from a medical perspective, and this has led to the sequestration of death and a lack of focus on the best methods to ensure that people, who will inherently die, are able to value death as a necessary component of the life span.

Many different types of professionals have recognized that there are distinct challenges in end-of-life decision-making that create challenges and can foster anxiety, fear, anger, and despair. In the study of clients seeking therapeutic support for addressing existential questions and seeking relief from death fear and death anxiety, the application of an existential psychoanalytic praxis provided some support for creating communication and social goals and fostering a sense of self-actualization. Generally, therapists found that they were more focused on the existential process for the elderly when applying the praxis and were able to address central issues, including death fear, death anxiety, and the pursuit of self-actualization. In contrast to this perspective, the data collected from interviews and a focus group suggested that there were some situations in which there were clear divisions on the approach and the best method to meet goals.

The data collected from interviews, the focus group, and survey materials for the therapists and clients at the facility reflect specific views of the approach, the ability to create a responsive relationship, and the ability to meet goals for addressing fundamental issues (Mason 357). The data reflects a division between the perspectives of some of the therapists on the best approaches to achieving goals and the varied views of clients about the success in applying the praxis to their therapeutic process. At the same time, the data also underscored perceived benefits of the existential psychoanalytic praxis in addressing some of the functional identified issues in end-of-life experiences.

This praxis has support in regard to specific challenges to the internal maturational plan and individuals face developmentally specific challenges that they must work through in a progression along the life span (Vail and Cavanaugh 41). Subsequently, the praxis provides support for a range of method of applying theoretical views of existential purpose and questioning to the evaluation of change that is inherent at the end of life. The implication of this research then is that it points to specific cumulative views of approaches that can be used to foster greater communication with people as they age and also suggests an inherent need for changes in the approaches to addressing self-actualization in aging populations.

❧ Summary

The truth of life is that it must end. Heidegger wrote, "One of these days one will die too, in the end; but right now it has nothing to do with us." The study presented embraces the existential view of the importance of death and the need to consider questions of mortality as essential to man's capacity to move through the life span. Heidegger's premise though maintains one of the struggles that is repeated throughout this research, and that is the belief that man struggles with the role that death plays.

The "medicalization" of death and the belief that it is something to be avoided drives research into the treatment of disease and creates a problem-based view of death as something that can be avoided for long periods of time. Even Heidegger's principle suggests that most people living in the world want to have very little to do with death and want to avoid it until it happens. This perspective has driven the case for the sequestration of death and for efforts to maintain life even in the presence of impending death and through the use of medically futile approaches.

The proposal of a therapeutic approach to addressing the death for aging populations facing end-of-life decision-making are components of this study, and the research supports the use of an existential psychoanalytic praxis. One of the key elements of this praxis is to reject the Rogerian view that questioning should not be used and instead seeks methods of supporting the asking of existential questions. At the same time, the foundation of the praxis is the existential views of Rogers, including the creation of a therapeutic relationship based on communication and trust through which a person can seek answers to questions of existence.

This research study not only defined a research foundation for the use of the praxis, but also assessed the use of the praxis in the therapeutic environment, assessing both the perspectives of therapists and of clients in regard to its application. This kind of research provides a foundational element for the application of the praxis and can be used for the creation of future research into praxis of this type. The approach, which focuses on the use of a mixed method data collection process and the identification of views from a varied population, was shaped by the belief that this information could serve to support a method of change.

One note that can be made in the research process is that there were some limitations in the application of information for supporting the praxis above all other approaches. First, the praxis was created as a culmination of approaches and so it is difficult to compare against commonly used approaches without some overlap. Second, the responses of the individuals were somewhat less than conclusive about the benefits of the praxis above other approaches, primarily because this as the first experience that some of the participants had in a therapeutic situation. Finally, the focus of the research is to create a foundation for the continued exploration of this kind of praxis.

In order to continue the exploration of praxis of this type, it is valuable to consider variations in the defining characteristics of the praxis or the foundational information used to determine the parameters. This research process provides a foundation and specific views that were developed as a part of the movement toward a completed approach, but they are not the only methods that can be used. The connection between different existential perspectives and ongoing research into the best methods to create a path toward self-actualization for aging adults is valuable to the field of psychology.

Future research in this field can include an exploration of other psychodynamic perspectives, the cultural and social views of death that impact psychological functioning for aging populations, and the creation of a novel view of self-actualization that more readily integrates different perspectives on the pursuit of the best sense of self possible. This future research is identified in the study and is reflective of the views of subjects reported through both interviews and the focus group. The study presented relates beneficial information for the treatment of aging adults in the therapeutic environment and promotes the asking of existential questions to ease the transition through the end of the life span.

APPENDIX A
ADMINISTRATIVE NEEDS
ASSESSMENT

Name of the Facility: _____

Address: _____

Number of Participants Enrolled in Therapy: _____

Administrator: _____

Reviewed by: _____ Date: _____

❊ Introduction

This rating scale will be distributed to two facilities for completion. The document will be directed to the administrator of each facility. The purpose of the rating scale is to assist facility personnel to improve the therapeutic response to the needs of elderly patients through an existential psychoanalytic praxis.

When properly guided and developed, this type of praxis is a purposeful part of a therapeutic process. It aids in the realization of objectives concerned with the development of through the life span, which can include identifying potential, pursuing self-actualization, developing meaning, and reducing death fear. The individual, to become a fully self-actualized individual, needs many opportunities to explore factors that can hinder self-actualization. To achieve this objective, the essentials of an existential psychoanalytic praxis need to be identified.

The rating scale is designed for self-appraisal by program/facility administrator.

❦ Use and Interpretation of the Scores

The rating scale is comprised of a series of ratings on the major areas that should concern facility personnel relative to psychotherapeutic programming for aging adults. There are six sections to the rating scale: consistency in approach, reducing fear, addressing self-actualization, and meeting client goals.

The rating score is on a scale from 0 to 4 with 0

meaning inadequate achievement and 4 meaning fully achieved with excellent results. Each section can be rated by the total section score and an overall rating can be obtained by totaling all sections of the rating scale. A careful analysis should be made of each statement, section, and overall rating to determine the areas in need of improvement. The interpretation of the score for each statement is the following:

0 – Inadequate/extremely limited

1 – Poor/exists but needs a great deal of improvement

2 – Fair/adequate but needs some improvement

3 – Good/well done and only needs periodic review

4 – Excellent/has achieved outstanding results

	Inadequate (0)	Poor (1)	Fair (2)	Good (3)	Excellent (4)
1. Do/does the current approach(es) used in the therapeutic environment support consistency and positive outcomes for clients and practitioners?					

2. Do/does the current approach(es) used in the therapeutic environment support death fear reduction?					
3. Do/does the current approach(es) used in the therapeutic environment address self-actualization as a goal of the therapeutic process?					
4. Do current psychotherapeutic approaches used in the facility meet the overarching needs of the client population?					

APPENDIX B
THE FOUNDATIONS
OF THE EXISTENTIAL
PSYCHOANALYTIC PRAXIS

The Threat to Dignity	Culturally Directed Quests	Existential Life Needs	Resolution through Existential Psychoanalysis
Death Fear	To be protected.	Courage to protect oneself.	Acceptance.
Death Anxiety	To be validated and honored.	Courage to pursue self-actualization.	Relief and nonengagement.
Guilt or Shame	To achieve.	Courage to obtain freedom from imperfection and insecurity.	Self-forgiveness.
Despair	To be safe and free from pain.	Courage to anticipate the meaning or actions of others.	Hope.
Helplessness	To be autonomous.	Courage to seek the support of others.	Trust and belief in others.

Loss of Self-Worth	To be valued.	Courage to value self above others.	Value.
Anger	To have an outlet for aggression.	Courage to transform experiences.	Joy.

APPENDIX C
IRB FORM

Each university provides standard IRB forms that must be utilized. The following is an example of an IRB form for consent to the use of human subject populations. You should receive a list of the IRB forms that you will have to include with your study.

http://www.uhhs.com/download/research/irb_form_consent_language_template_92002b.rtf

❈ Summary of Your Rights as a Participant in a Research Study

Your participation in this research study is voluntary. Refusing to participate in the study will not have a negative impact. If you decide to join the study, you may withdraw at any time and for any reason without penalty.

If information generated from this study is published or presented, your identity will not be revealed. In the event new information becomes available that may affect the risks or benefits associated with this study or your willingness to participate in it, you will be notified so that you can decide whether or not to continue participating.

✖ Disclosure of Your Study Records

Efforts will be made to keep the personal information in your research record private and confidential, but absolute confidentiality cannot be guaranteed. The Institutional Review Board may review your study records. If your records are reviewed, your identity could become known.

✖ Contact Information

_____ has described to you what is going to be done, including the risks, hazards, and benefits involved, and can be contacted at _____.

Signature _____

Signing below indicates that you have been informed about the research study in which you voluntarily agree to participate, that you have asked any questions about the study that you may have, and that the information given to you has permitted you to make a fully informed and free decision about your participation in the study. By signing this consent form, you do not waive any legal rights, and the investigator(s) or sponsor(s) are not relieved of any liability they may have. A copy of this consent form will be provided to you.

[Add the appropriate signature block from the choices below. Do not start the signature block on a new page unless this page is full.]

[Signature format for studies enrolling only adults.]

_____ Date_____

 Signature of Participant

_____

 Printed Name of Participant

_____ Date_____

Signature of Person Obtaining Consent

_____

Printed Name of Person Obtaining Consent

(Must be study investigator or individual who has been designated in the checklist to obtain consent.)

_____ Date_____

Signature of Principal Investigator
(affirming subject eligibility for the
study and that informed consent has
been obtained)

(Revised 09/2002)

APPENDIX D
PERSONAL QUESTIONNAIRE

Subject #_____

Demographic Information

Subject Age_____

Gender_____

Please select the term that best describes your ethnicity:

1) Anglo European White
2) Afro African, Afro Caribbean, or African American
3) Hispanic
4) Asian or Pacific Islander
5) Native American
6) Other

Please select the term that best describes your socioeconomic status:

1) Lower
2) Middle
3) Upper

What was the last year of school you completed?

1) Middle school or less (eighth grade)
2) Some high school
3) High school diploma
4) Some college
5) Undergraduate degree
6) Graduate degree or greater

Please answer the following questions with yes or no.
Are you a therapist?
Are you a client? If yes, are you currently seeking the support of a therapist?

Is there anything else you would like us to know?

APPENDIX E
RESEARCH SUBJECT INFORMED CONSENT FORM FOR INTERVIEW AND FOCUS GROUP PARTICIPANTS

Prospective Research Subject: Please read the following consent form before determining your willingness to participate in the study.

(The student must fill in the following specific information to complete the informed consent form based on this example paper.)

Project information:
Project title:
Project number:
Sponsor:
Principal investigator:
Organization:
Location:
Phone:

❋ Purpose of This Research Study

The purpose of this study is to assess the use of an existential psychoanalytic praxis for the treatment of elderly clients. This study will evaluate the views of both clients and therapists regarding the benefits or limitations of this type of approach in addressing death fear, death anxiety, and self-actualization.

❋ Procedures

Participants will be asked to complete two questionnaires, one with demographic characteristics and the other representing their views on specific issues. Some participants will be asked to be a part of a focus group, and others will be interviewed.

❋ Ownership and Documentation

The responses and data collected will become the possession of the researcher and will be used to create a narrative document reflecting the outcomes of the subject population. The entire responses to demographic information will not be included in the final research document but used to assess variations in outcomes related to the approach utilized and the variables identified.

✳ Possible Benefits

The outcomes of this study will be provided to organizations to demonstrate the value of the use of an existential psychoanalytic praxis in the outpatient setting. This will relate to the views of both therapists and clients.

✳ Confidentiality

Your identity, including name, identification number, and identifying conditions, will not be related at any point in the study. The researchers will maintain a strict code of confidentiality, and no personal information will be discussed or divulged in any manner outside the scope of the study outcomes. The subject's name, identifying characteristics, comments, or additional information will not be discussed outside the research team.

❧ Termination of Participation

You are free to choose not to participate in this research study. Even after completing this document, you can choose at any point to terminate your participation.

❧ Available Sources of Information

Any further questions you have about this study will be answered by the Principal Investigator.

Name:
Phone number:

❧ Authorization

I have read and understand this consent form, and I volunteer to participate in this research study. I understand that I will receive a copy of this form. I voluntarily choose to participate, but I understand that my consent does not take away any legal rights in the case of negligence or other legal fault of anyone who is involved in this study. I further understand that nothing in this consent form is intended to replace any applicable national, state, or local laws.

Participant name (printed or typed):

Date:

Principal investigator signature:

Date:

APPENDIX F
INTERVIEW AND FOCUS
GROUP QUESTIONS

❋ Interview Questions

What are the approaches you commonly use to explore issues of death fear or death anxiety in elderly populations?

What are the most significant barriers to effective treatment of elderly patients with end-of-life issues?

What are your views on the effectiveness of the existential psychoanalytic praxis presented?

Can you describe any difference in the response to the approach as compared to the approaches you more commonly use with your clients?

Can you identify any areas of improvement for the praxis?

Are there specific strategies that work better than others in supporting the exploration of self-actualization in elderly populations?

❊ Focus Groups Questions

What are the main characteristics of an effective therapist when addressing issues in end-of-life planning?

What are you looking for in therapy in terms of your fears, anxieties, or expectations?

Have you experienced any benefits from your therapist using the new existential praxis?

How effective is your therapist in providing the support you need to address concerns about end-of-life experiences?

Do you believe that your experiences in therapy have helped you address concerns you have about the meaningfulness of your life?

Can you discuss any improvements to the praxis that has been introduced?

APPENDIX G
EXAMPLE TRANSCRIPTION
FROM FOCUS GROUP

Table 1

For the purpose of this narrative, participants who spoke were identified with numbers that included codes for gender and age. For example, a sixty-two-year-old participant would be identified as P1-F62 (Participant 1, Female, Age 62). The facilitator is identified simply as F.

F: Thank you all for joining me for this focus group. The purpose of this group is to ask you some questions about your work with your therapist in recent months and to provide an opportunity for you to discuss your views among yourselves. Just so I'm sure you are all aware, we are recording this information and will be transcribing it for our study. OK. So our first question is this: What are the main characteristics of an effective therapist when addressing issues in end-of-life planning?

[Silence]

P1-F82: I'm not sure what you mean.

F: Well, what would you say are the things that make your therapist or another therapist effective in their job?

P1-F82: This might seem obvious, but they have to be good communicators. I mean, I can tell when someone isn't a good therapist. You know, he asks questions but doesn't really say what he means, or I'm not really sure what he's asking. Sometimes he tries to hide what he's asking by asking it in a complicated way. And sometimes what's important to him is not important to me, so he doesn't address my issues.

P2-F74: I know what you mean. A good therapist has to talk about what I need to talk about, not some other stuff. Sometimes I think it must be obvious what's bothering me. I guess he's good if he knows I'm struggling and asks about it.

F: What else?

P3-M73: I like when he gives it to me straight. I don't really want to have to talk around things for the whole time.

P4-M77: Yeah, but sometimes I'm glad when he knows I don't want to talk about things, but he pushes me because that's what we're doing here.

P1-F82: Well, it's always good if he reminds me why I'm here. I can't always remember.

P4-M77: That's about right.

P3-M73: Well, you talk all the time anyway, [Bob]. I can't imagine a time when you don't just spill your guts. If the guy's listening, you probably figure he's good.

P4-M77. Yup.

F: Any other things you think make a good therapist? How about someone who hasn't spoken yet?

P5-F80: Two weeks ago, we sat down and started a new process. It was about setting some goals that I could achieve and talking about ways of reaching those goals. For example, one of my goals was to reconcile with my daughter. My therapist asked if I would frame that in terms of my end-of-life experiences and so I told him that I wanted to reconcile with my daughter before I died. When I said it out loud, I realized that he was helping me to understand the need for this kind of change. With goals, I can know where we're going each time.

P4-M77: I can see how that would be a good thing. I think communication is key, again. I need to hear what it is we're doing and why, and I need to have the situation be clear. There is no room in my life for a therapist who is wishy-washy. I don't have that kind of time.

P6-F69: I hate when you talk that way. You're always bringing up the time thing. I just want to let it go. Stop thinking about it so much.

[Silence]

F: OK, let's try another question. What are you looking for in therapy in terms of your fears, anxieties, or expectations?

[Silence]

F: Any thoughts?

P4-M77: I hate talking about this stuff in therapy. I don't really want to talk about it with you too.

F: Well, we're talking about it to see if we can make changes to your therapy process that would help you.

P4-M77: I'm not an idiot, you know. I know why you're here. If we're being frank—

P3-M73: You're always frank. We're trying to talk here.

P4-M77: Don't need to pipe in. If we're being frank, my biggest issue is fear. Sometimes my fear is debilitating and I can't even get out of bed. It's constant.

P5-F80: Fear, yeah, but I also feel like I lack control in my life. If I can't be in control in my final days, what should I be in control of? I don't know. I just feel helpless.

P1-F82: I think the biggest part of my anxiety comes from not knowing what to expect and not knowing how I can be in control. I think that's why I turn to God. I'm hoping he's going to figure it out for me.

P4-M77: All I know is when your time is up, your time is up, and when it's over, it's over. I'm bothered by the finality of it all.

P5-F80: I can't really get my mind around it. My daughter keeps pushing me to figure out what to do about my health issues because I think she's more afraid of it than I am. My anxiety comes out of all the pressure to solve the issues. I mean, really, death is the end, and sometimes it has to happen. I feel both fear and anxiety, but for the most part, I feel a lot of shame over being afraid. I keep thinking it shouldn't be this hard.

P4-M77: That's because you're lacking faith in an afterlife. If you believed in God fully, you'd be able to see the end as a positive thing.

P7-F79: You're full of it! No one wants to see death as a positive thing. No one sees it that way. I love God and all, but I'm not going to give up the fight just because he's up there.

F: Anyone have any different thoughts about your expectations about therapy?

P8-F77: I'm hoping to continue working on some of my issues with my family. It shouldn't be this hard. I keep telling them I want to be involved in the decision-making process, but they don't see that as important.

P9-F89: I mean they do it for people who are dying from disease; everyone wants to be on their support team. I watched a friend's daughter go through her breast cancer and all of her family members and coworkers got behind her, even though she eventually died. I liked that view. I would love to feel part of a team that supported my choices. My family just can't hear it, so I guess my expectation is to improve communication.

P10-F88: Your team? Really? I would rather just have help with end-of-life choices and feel that my family and I could share expectations. I'd like to feel in control of that situation, and maybe they could provide feedback but not always try to change the choices I've made.

P11-M81: If you're like me, as soon as you show any weakness, they try to take everything away. As soon as I stopped being able to do everything for myself, they stopped wanting me involved in the decision-making process. I don't want to lose my faculties and have them just go nuts making decisions I never would have made. I hate the idea of the humiliation of it all.

P12-M90: It's really complicated, but my anxiety comes from feeling humiliated and having people do everything for me.

[Silence]

F: How about another question? A few months ago, your therapists discussed with you using a new approach that focused on some of these central existential questions and also helped you focus on specific elements and conflicts that come out of your experiences. Have you experienced any benefits from your therapist using the new existential praxis?

P13-F75: My therapist seemed unsure of what she was doing at first, and I thought that maybe she just wasn't prepared.

P9-F89: I know what you mean.

P4-M77: There was a difference in the level of experience with this approach and others.

P1-F82: I don't know what you mean by that. I think unsure is a better word for it.

P12-M90: I've seen this before. Sometimes when they are told to do things a certain way, they don't have the willingness to implement change. That's a fancy way of saying that they resisted the new way of doing things.

P1-F82: Maybe they just needed more training.

P12-M90: Maybe. Or maybe they were just less comfortable and kept falling back on the traditional approach.

P1–F82: I thought it was interesting to be doing things a new way. I liked the change. It was good to see a connection between my personal goals and the results.

F: Were you able to see those connections?

P1–F82: I felt like the new system gave me some feedback and ways of looking at things that was helpful.

P5–F80: I felt like we got past some stuff. I mean, it was good that he didn't seem so stuck in his ways. Funny coming from me, huh?

P4–M77: Yup. I don't know. I felt like he did a good job, but sometimes I don't want to always have to change.

P6–F69: See, and I felt like my therapist didn't want to use the new systems, so she didn't.

F: Last question: How effective is your therapist in providing the support you need to address concerns about end-of-life experiences?

P4–M77: I think we got started, but we need to continue. There's more to do.

P3-M73: I agree. You know, my therapist described one of the parts of this approach as getting beneficial outcomes related to goals. I think that's my approach. I think I'm still working on it.

P4-M77: I agree.

P5-F80: I don't like the way we talk about things. I don't like the term "end-of-life planning." It's not helpful.

P1-F82: I agree. I also don't like when they talk about elderly care needs as if they are separate from anyone else's care needs.

P4-M77: That's because you're independent right now. It may not always be that way.

P5-F80: I think there are better ways to frame this information.

P4-M77: You sound like a therapist.

P5-F80. I know. I hate the way it sounds.

F: Let's be more specific. Do you believe that your experiences in therapy have helped you address concerns you have about the meaningfulness of your life?

P4-M77: We've got more to do. I'm a work in progress, you know.

P1-F82: You always say things like that. I'm not sure how we're supposed to figure out if it's meaningful. I mean, I feel better talking about things, but I'm not sure if I would describe it as meaningful. I'm not sure I'll know if its meaningful until it's over.

P4-M77: What do you mean by "it's over"? Life or therapy.

P1-F82: Life.

P12-M90: I don't know about that, but I keep telling my stories when people will listen. I want to be remembered.

P1-F82: That's the hardest part about this. I feel like I'm struggling to figure out if I just want to be remembered or if I'm having a hard time because it has gone by too fast.

P12-M90: You know what they say: time is wasted on the young. If I only knew what I know now when I was a kid, I wouldn't have wasted so much time.

P5-F80: I agree.

REFERENCES

Administration on Aging. "Aging Statistics," United States Department of Health and Human Services, 2014.

Ahlzen, R. (2011). Illness as unhomelike being-in-the-world? Phenomenology and Medical Practice. Medicine and Health Care Philosophy, 14(3), 323–331.

Albanese, J. *Professional Ethics in Criminal Justice: Being Ethical When No One Is Looking.* Upper Saddle River, NJ: Pearson Education, Inc., 2012.

Allport, G. "Concepts of Trait and Personality." *Psychological Bulletin,* 24 (1927): 284–293.

Allport, G. "Functional Autonomy of Motives." *The American Journal of Psychology,* 50 (1937): 141–156.

Aristotle. *The Nicomachean Ethics.* Harmondsworth: Penguin, 1976.

Barrett, W. H. *Irrational Man: A Study in Existential Philosophy.* New York: Doubleday, 1958.

Battin, Margaret P. "The Concept of Rational Suicide." In Edwin S. Shneidman, ed., Death: Current Perspectives. Palo Alto, CA: Mayfield Publishing Company, 1984.

Beach, M. C. and Morrison, S. R. "The effect of do-not-resuscitate orders on physician decision-making." Journal of the American Geriatrics Society, 50.12 (2002): 2057–2062.

Berg, C., Meegan, S., and Deviney, F. A social-context model of coping with everyday problems across the lifespan. International Journal of Behavioral Development, 22.2 (1998): 239–261.

Berger, K. S. The Developing Person through the Life Span. New York: Worth Publishing, 2004.

Birren, J. E. and Deutchman, D. Guiding Autobiography Groups for Older Adults: Exploring the Fabric of Life. Baltimore: The Johns Hopkins University Press, 1991.

Boeree, C. G. "Abraham Maslow." 2006. Web. 5 October 2014.

Bradby, Hannah (2012). Medicine, Health, and Society. Los Angeles, CA: Sage Publications.

Butler, R. N. "Life Review: An Interpretation of Reminiscence in the Aged." Psychiatry 4 (1963): 1–8.

Butler, R. N. "Age: The Life-review." Psychology Today 7 (1971): 49–51.

Butler, R. N. (1974). "Successful aging and the role of Life Review." Journal of the American Geriatrics Society 22 (1974): 529–535.

Butts, J. and Rich, K. "Rational suicide: uncertain moral ground." Journal of Advanced Nursing, 46.3 (2004): 270–278.

Capuzzi, C. and Gross, D. Counseling and Psychotherapy: Theories and Interventions, 4th ed. Upper Saddle River, NJ: Prentice Hall, 2004.

Casper, J. Forests: More than Just Trees. Infobase Publishing, 2007.

Centers for Disease Control and Prevention. "The State of Mental Health and Aging in America," 2014.

Choron, J. Modern Man and Mortality. New York: Macmillan, 1964.

Collett, L. and Lester, D. "The Fear of Death and Fear of Dying," Journal of Psychology 72 (1969): 179–181.

Conway, S. Governing Death and Loss. London: Oxford University Press, 2010.

Cooper, M. "Therapists' experiences of relational depth: A qualitative interview study." Counseling and Psychotherapy Research, 5.2 (2005): 87–95.

Cooper, M. Essential Research Findings in Counseling and Psychotherapy: The Facts are Friendly. London: Sage Publications, 2008.

Cooper, M. "Relational depth: Where we are now." Presentation given at the 2nd relational depth conference: Relational depth: Current theory and practice, University of Nottingham, July 1, 2009.

Curtis, J. and Burt, R. "Futility in the intensive care unit: Hard cases make bad law." Critical Care Medicine, 38.8 (2010): 1742–1743.

Corey, G. Theory and Practice of Counseling and Psychotherapy, 8th ed. Publisher: Thomson Brooks/Cole, 2008.

Creswell, J. Research Design: Qualitative, Quantitative and Mixed Methods Approaches, 2nd ed. Thousand Oaks, CA: Sage, 2003.

Curran, Charles E. "The Catholic Moral Tradition in Bioethics" in Walter, Jennifer and Eran P. Klein, eds. The Story of Bioethics: From seminal works to contemporary explorations Georgetown University Press, 2003.

Delongis, A. and Holtzman, S. Coping in context: the role of stress, social support, and personality in coping. Journal of Personality, 73.6(2006): 1633–1656.

Erikson's Stages of Development. 2010.

Erskine, R., Moursund, J., and Trautmann, R. Beyond Empathy: A Therapy of Contact-in-Relationship. Washington, DC: Psychology Press, 1999.

Farber, B. "On the enduring and substantial influence of Carl Rogers's not-quite necessary nor sufficient conditions." Psychotherapy: Theory, Research, Practice, Training, 44.3 (2007): 289–294.

Feifel, H., and Branscomb, A. B. "Who's Afraid of Death?" Journal of Abnormal Psychology, 81 (1973): 282–288.

Feifel, H., and Nagy, V. T. "Another look at fear of death." Journal of Consulting and Clinical Psychology, 49 (1981): 278–286.

Feist, J. and Feist, G. Theories of Personality (7th ed.). New York: McGraw Hill, 2009.

Frankl, V. Man's Search for Meaning, Part One, "Experiences in a Concentration Camp." New York: Pocket Books.

Freud, S. Uncanny (trans. David McLintock). London: Penguin Books, 1919.

Freud, S., Freud, F., and Strachey, J. The Essentials of Psychoanalysis. Harmondsworth: Penguin, 1991.

Frie, R. "Subjectivity and Intersubjectivity in Modern Philosophy and Psychoanalysis. Lanhman, Maryland: Rowman and Littlefield Publishers, Inc., 1997.

Galeni Opera Omnia. Basel: Par'Andrea to Kratandro, 1538.Kühn, C. G. Galeni Opera Omnia. Leipzig: C. Cnobloch, 1821–1833, rpt.

Internet Encyclopedia of Philosophy. "Galen 130–200 C.E." https://iep.utm.edu/galen/.

Garcia-Ballester, L. (2002) Galen and Galenism: Theory of medical practice from antiquity to the European Renaissance. Jon Arrizabalaga, Montserrat Cabre, Lluis Cifuentes, and Fernando Salmon (Eds.). Variorum Collected Studies Series. Aldershot, UK: Ashgate.

Greenberg, L. and Geller, S. "Congruence and therapeutic presence," (2001): 148–166.

Grogan, J. "Cultural History of the Humanistic Psychology Movement in America." The University of Texas at Austin. UMI No. 3311487. Ann Arbor, MI: ProQuest, LLC, 2008.

Hachler, N. (2013). Galen's observations on disease of the soul and the mind of men-Researches on the knowledge of mental illness in antiquity. Rosetta, 13, 53–72.

Haynes, C. "Ethics in End of Life Care." Journal of Hospice and Palliative Nursing, 6(2004): 36.

Heidegger, M. (1977). The Question Concerning Technology. In The Question Concerning Technology and Other Essays, trans. William Lovitt. New York: Garland Publishing.

Heidegger, Martin. *Being and Time.* San Francisco: Harper Collins, 1962.

Holme, R. Psychology Today. Del Mar, CA: CRM Books, 1972.

Illich, I. (1976). Medical nemesis: The exploration of health. New York: Random House.

Kirschenbaum, H. "Carl Rogers's life and work: an assessment on the 100th anniversary of his birth." Journal of Counseling & Development 82(2004): 116–124.

Klug, L., and Boss, M. "Further study of the validity of the death concern scale." Psychological Report 40 (1977): 907–910.

Klug, L., and Sinha, A. "Death acceptance: A two-component formulation and scale." Omega 18(1987): 229–235.

Knox, R. and Cooper, Mick. "A state of readiness: an exploration of the client's role in meeting at relational depth." Journal of Humanistic Psychology, 51.1 (2011): 61–81.

Kolden, G., Klein, M. H., Wang, C., and Austin, S. B. "Congruence/Genuineness." In J. C. Norcross (Ed.), Psychotherapy Relationships That Work (2nd ed.). New York: Oxford University Press, 2011.

Krell, D. Martin Heidegger: Basic Writings. San Francisco: Harper Collins, 1993.

Langle, A. and Probst, C. Existential questions of the elderly. International Medical Journal, 7.3 (2000): 193–196.

Laureate Education, Inc. Coping in a social context. 2012. Unpublished document.

Lee, Patrick. "Human beings are animals. International Philosophical Quarterly 37 (1997): 291–303.

Lehoux, P. (2006). "The Problem of Health Technology: Policy Implications for Modern Health Care Systems. CRC Press.

Malette, J. and Oliver, L. "Retirement and existential meaning in the older adult: A qualitative study using life review. Counseling, Psychotherapy, and Health, 2.1 (2006): 30–49.

Maslow, A. H. "A Theory of Metamotivation : The Biological Rooting of the Value-Life." Journal of Humanistic Psychology 7.2 (1967): 93–127.

Mason, M. Rogers redux: Relevance and outcomes of motivational interviewing across behavioral problems. Journal of Counseling & Development, 87.3 (2009): 357–363.

May, R., and Yalom, I. "Existential Psychotherapy." In R. J. Corsini and D. Wedding (Eds.). Current Psychotherapies (4th ed.). Itasca, IL: F. E. Peacock Publishers, Inc., 1989.

May, R. (1977). The meaning of anxiety (rev. ed.). New York: Norton.

McKenzie, H. "Personal and Collective Fears of Death," In Fagan, A. (Ed). Making Sense of Dying and Death. Rodopi, 2004.

McNamara, B. Fragile Lives: Death, Dying and Care. Buckingham: Open University Press, 2001.

Mearns, D., and Thorne, B. Person-centered Counseling in Action. London, UK: Sage, 2007.

Mellor, P. and Shilling, C. "Modernity, self identity and the sequestration of death. Sociology 27.3 (1993): 411–431.

Merleau-Ponty, M. Phenomenology of Perception. (C. Smith, Trans.). London: Routledge, 1962.

Orr, R. D. "Pain management rather than assisted suicide: the ethical high ground." Pain Medicine 2 (2001): 2–10.

Pearce, W. B. "Trust in interpersonal relationships." Speech Monographs, 41 (1974): 236–244.

Plato. (1968). Republic. Trans., Alan Bloom. New York: Basic Books.

Plato. (1969). Laws. A. E. Taylor, Trans. Collected Dialogues of Plato. E. Hamilton and H. Cairns, Ed. Princeton: Princeton University Press.

Rodin, M. P. "Non-engagement, failure to engage and disengagement." In Duck, S. (Ed). Personal relationships, 4: Dissolving personal relationships. New York: Academic Press, 1982.

Rogers, C. Carl Rogers on Personal Power. NY: Delacorte Press, 1977.

Rogers, C. Client-centered Therapy: Its Current Practice, Implications and Theory. London: Constable, 1951.

Rogers, C., Gendlin, E. T., Kiesler, D. J., and Truax, C. B. (Eds.). The therapeutic relationship and its impact: A study of psychotherapy with schizophrenics. Madison, WI: University of Wisconsin Press, 1967.

Rogers, C. *A Way of Being.* New York: Houghton Mifflin, 1955.

Rogers, C. and Sanford, R. C. Client-centered psychotherapy. In H. I. Kaplan and B. J. Sadock (Eds.), Comprehensive textbook of psychiatry, IV. Baltimore: Williams and Wilkins, 1984.

Rogers, C. Significant aspects of client-centered therapy. American Psychologists, 1 (1946): 415–422.

Rogers, C. A Theory of Therapy, Personality and Interpersonal Relationships as Developed in the Client-centered Framework. In (ed.) S. Koch, Psychology: A Study of a Science. Vol. 3: Formulations of the Person and the Social Context. New York: McGraw Hill, 1959.

Remler, D. and Van Ryzin, G. Research Methods in Practice. Los Angeles: Sage, 2011.

Rich, B. "Causation and Intent: Persistent Conundrums in End-of-Life Care." Cambridge Quarterly of Healthcare Ethics, 16 (2007): 63–73.

Roberts, D. (2011). Philosophy and Science Fiction. Retrieved from http://introductiontophilosophy.com/chap6f.html

Sartre, J. P. Existential Psychoanalysis. (H. E. Barnes, Trans). Washington, DC: Gateway Edition, 1962.

Savin-Baden, M. and Major, C. Qualitative Research: The Essential Guide to Theory and Practice. London: Routledge, 2013.

Schrag, Zachary M. "Behind Closed Doors: IRBs and the Making of Ethical Research," American Journal of Sociology 118 (2012): 494–496.

Schneiderman, L. "Defining medical futility and improving medical care." Journal of Bioethical Inquiry, 8(2011): 123–131.

Socrates. "Apology." 2000.

Stanley, L. and Wise, S. "The Domestication of Death: The Sequestration Thesis and Domestic Figuration." Sociology 45(2011): 947–962.

Strine, T., Chapman, D., Balluz, L., and Mokdad, A. "Health-related Quality of Life and Health Behaviors by Social and Emotional Support: Their Relevance to Psychiatry and Medicine," Social Psychiatry and Psychiatric Epidemiology 43(2008): 151–159.

Svenaeus, S. (2010). The hermeneutics of medicine and the phenomenology of health; Steps towards a philosophy of medical practice. Norwell, MA: Kluwer Academic Publishers.

Tauber, Alfred I. Patient Autonomy and the Ethics of Responsibility. Cambridge: MIT Press, 2005.

Topfer, F. and Wiesing, U. (2005). The medical theory of Richard Koch I: Theory of science and ethics. Medical and Health Care Philosophy, 8(2), 207–219.

Vincent, S. Being Empathic: A Companion for Counselors and Therapists. Milton Keynes, UK: Radcliffe Publishing, 2005.

Thomas, J. Comprehensive Handbook of Personality and Psychopathology, Volume 1. Hoboken, NJ: John Wiley and Sons, 2006.

Trusty, Jerry, Ng, Kok-Mun and Watts, Richard E. "Model of effects of adult attachment on emotional empathy of counseling students." Journal of Counseling and Development 83(2005): 66.

Vail, R. and Cavanaugh, J. Human Development: A Lifespan View, 5th ed. Belmont, CA: Wadsworth, 2010.

Walter, T. "Modern death: taboo or not taboo?" Sociology 25.2 (1991): 293 –310.

Whelton, W. J. and Greenberg, L. S. "Psychological Contact and Perception as Dialogical Construction. In P. Sanders and G. Wyatt (Eds.), Rogers's Therapeutic Conditions. Volume 4: Contact and Perception. Ross-On-Wye: PCCS Books, 2001.

Willmott, H. "Death. So what? Sociology, Sequestration and Emancipation," The Sociological Review 48(2000): 649–665.

Yalom, I. Existential Psychotherapy. New York: Basic Books, 1981.

Yalom, I. "Staring at the Sun: Overcoming the Terror of Death." The Humanistic Psychologist, 36.3 (2008): 283–297.

AMA. (2018). *AMA Principles of Medical Ethics.* Retrieved from the American Medical Association. https://www.ama-assn.org/delivering-care/ama-principles-medical-ethics.

AMA. (n.d.). *History of the Code.* Retrieved from the American Medical Association. ama-code-ethics-history.pdf.

Daniel, M. (2016, May 3). *Study Suggests Medical Errors Now Third Leading Cause of Death in US. Physicians Advocate for Changes in How Deaths are Reported to Better Reflect Reality.* Retrieved from Johns Hopkins Medicine. https://www.hopkinsmedicine.org/news/media/releases/study_suggests_medical_errors_now_third_leading_cause_of_death_in_the_us.

Dell'Oro, R. (2016. June). Why Clinical Ethics? Experience, Discernment and the Anamnesis of Meaning at the Bedside. *Persona y Bioetica, 20*(1), 86–98.

Devoe, D. (2012). Viktor Frankl's Logotherapy: The Search for Purpose and Meaning. *Inquiries Journal, 4*(7), 1–31.

Duffy, J. (2004). Rediscovering the Meaning in Medicine: Lessons from the Dying on the Ethics of Experience. *Palliative & Supportive Care, 2*(2), 207–211.

Frankl, V. E. (1962). *The Will to Meaning.* Retrieved from Panarchy. https://www.panarchy.org/index.html.

Peel, M. (2005, April). Human Rights and Medical Ethics. *Journal of the Royal Society of Medicine, 98*(4), 171–173.

Pennock, S. F. (2016, February 6). *On the Meaning of Meaning: What Are We Really Looking For?* Retrieved from the Positive Psychology Program. https://positivepsychologyprogram.com/meaning/.

Spriggs, M. (1998). Autonomy in the face of a Devastating Diagnosis. *Journal of Medical Ethics, 24*, 123–126.

Veatch, R. M. (2006). How Philosophy of Medicine has Changed Medical Ethics. *Journal of Medicine and Philosophy, 31*(6),

Wong, P. (2014, April 26). Viktor Frankl's Meaning-Seeking Model and Positive Psychology. *Positive Living Newsletter.* Retrieved from http://www.drpaulwong.com/viktor-frankls-meaning-seeking-model-and-positive-psychology/.

Wong, P. and Reilly, T. (2017, August 15). *Frankl's Self-Transcendence Model and Virtue Ethics.* Retrieved from Notre Dame. http://www.drpaulwong.com/frankls-self-transcendence-model-and-virtue-ethics/.

INDEX

B

Barrett, William, 24–25
The Belmont Report, 17–18
beneficence
  defined, 12
  principle of, xxx, xxxi
Binswanger, Ludwig, 26, 30, 33
biology, as a science, xiii
biology-focused approach, to coping
  with aging, 57, 58
Birren, J. E., 111, 113
Boss, M., 63
Butler, R. N., 111, 113

C

"Causation and Intent: Persistent
  Conundrums in End-of-Life
  Care" (Rich), 7–8
CEJA (Council on Ethical and
  Judicial Affairs), xxi
Centers for Disease Control and
  Prevention (CDC)
  on anxiety as underreported, 15
  on mental health issues in current
    aging population, 14
  report on medical errors causing
    deaths, xxxviii
cognitive impairment, as mental
  health concern of elderly, 15
communication
  as important element in
    therapeutic model, 127, 134,
    135, 136, 139
  lack of trust in, 137
conceptual gestalt, 50
conflicts, in therapeutic
  relationship, 138
congruence

according to Rogers, 52, 59
  as most difficult condition for
    therapists to realize, 134
Conway, S., 105–106
Cooper, M., 60
Council on Ethical and Judicial
  Affairs (CEJA), xxi
culture
  as defining way we view
    death, 101
  exploration of in therapeutic
    setting, 126
  influence of on therapeutic
    presence, 140

D

Darwin, Charles, xxxviii, xxxix
Dasein, 27, 28, 34
Dawkins, Richard, xxxviii
death. *See also* dying
  addressing of from new existential
    psychoanalytical approach,
    101–102, 111, 112. *See also*
    existential psychoanalytical
    praxis
  as boundary situation, 16
  as concern in end-of-life
    experiences, 3
  conflicting views on, 63–65
  culture as defining way we
    view, 101
  as enigmatic enemy, 102
  inevitability of, 5, 8, 34, 117, 124
  lack of understanding of value
    of, 7
  legitimization of, 124
  medical technologies as waylaying,
    4, 8, 64–65, 115, 117, 120
  medicalization of, 103

Illich, Ivan, xii
illness, negative stigmatization of, 5
incongruence, according to Rogers, 47, 53–54, 55
informed consent
  form, 163–167
  as issue of medical ethics, xxix
institutions, use of to create structure for death, 6–7, 8, 65, 102
interview questions, 169–170
IRB form, 157–160
isolation, as concern in end-of-life experiences, 3

J

Johns Hopkins, xxxvii–xxxviii
Jung, Carl, 2, 24, 30, 40–41
justice, principle of, xxx, xxxi

K

Kafka, Franz, 26
Kant, Immanuel, xxiii, xxvi, xxix
Kass, Leon, xxxi, xxxii
Kierkegaard, Soren, 26
Klug, L., 63
Knox, L., 60

L

Langle, A., 107, 108, 110, 112
Leviathan (Hobbes), xx
life
  should individuals live past their ability to sustain their own lives? 142
  variables in how individuals perceive progress of, 124–125
life-prolonging technologies, 142
life-sustaining technologies, 145

literature, analytical review of, 22–66
lived body, as distinct from physical body, xiv
living wills, 142
Locke, John, xxix
logotherapy, xxxiii

M

Maslow, Abraham, 2, 24, 36–38, 40, 117, 121–123, 127, 140, 141
May, Rollo, 2, 10, 24, 26, 35–36, 37, 62, 117, 123
meaning
  can it be retrieved, xxxiv–xxxvii
  of meaning, xxi–xxii
  suspension of, xxvii–xxviii
meaningfulness, shift in views on, 3
meaninglessness, as concern in end-of-life experiences, 3
medical community, focus of a half century ago, 141–142
medical errors, as third leading cause of death in US, xxxvii–xxxviii
medical ethics
  changes in, xxii–xxvi
  defined, xix–xlii
  overview/history of, xxviii–xxxiv
  what would happen if medical ethical codes were eliminated, xxxvii–xlii
medical futility, 144, 145
medical history, taking of for patient, xvi
medical technology
  burgeoning of, 141–142
  consequences of changes in, 4
  desire to advance, 143

www.ingramcontent.com/pod-product-compliance
Lightning Source LLC
Chambersburg PA
CBHW021356210526
45463CB00001B/114